Odon NSWELE ILUNDU

Fundamentals of Epidemiology

Odon NSWELE ILUNDU

Fundamentals of Epidemiology

Concepts, Causality and Practices

ScienciaScripts

Cover image: www.ingimage.com

This book is a translation from the original published under ISBN 978-3-639-65370-0.

Publisher:
Sciencia Scripts
is a trademark of
Dodo Books Indian Ocean Ltd. and OmniScriptum S.R.L publishing group

120 High Road, East Finchley, London, N2 9ED, United Kingdom
Str. Armeneasca 28/1, office 1, Chisinau MD-2012, Republic of Moldova, Europe
Managing Directors: Ieva Konstantinova, Victoria Ursu
info@omniscriptum.com

Printed at: see last page
ISBN: 978-620-8-39800-2

SUMMARY

This book explores the fundamental principles of epidemiology, providing a comprehensive foundation for understanding essential concepts, causal relationships and practices in epidemiology. It is aimed at students, researchers and public health practitioners who wish to deepen their knowledge of epidemiological methods and their application in a variety of settings. Focusing on theoretical foundations, analysis of causality and integration of practices, this book guides the reader through the evolution of the discipline and contemporary challenges.

This book presents the fundamental principles of epidemiology: Concepts, Causality and Practice. It is structured as follows:

- *Chapter 1 describes the basic concepts of epidemiology;*
- *The second chapter deals with statistical association and the notion of causality;*
- *The third chapter deals with prevention and screening;*
- *The fourth chapter announces the epidemiological studies;*
- *The fifth chapter presents measures of disease frequency;*
- *The sixth chapter deals with the measurement of association in epidemiology;*
- *Chapter seven outlines the investigation of epidemics and epidemiological surveillance;*
- *Chapter eight deals with sampling.*

FOREWORD

Epidemiology is a key discipline for understanding and preventing disease in populations. Although the foundations of epidemiology were laid centuries ago, its concepts and methods continue to evolve with scientific and technological advances. This book aims to bridge the gap between theory and practice, exploring founding principles and modern approaches. We hope it will inspire readers to use this knowledge to improve public health and enhance disease prevention.

BIBLIOGRAPHY

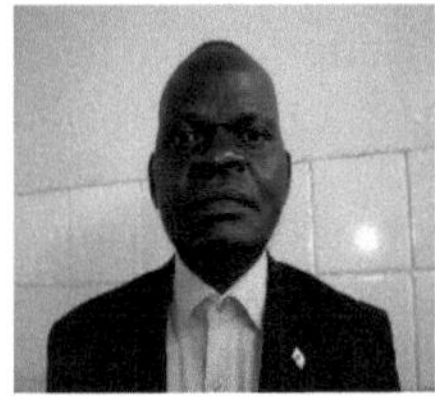

NSWELE ILUNDU Odon holds a Master 120 (Master 2) degree in Public Health, specializing in Community Health Policies and Programs, from the Université Catholique de Louvain (U.C.L) in Belgium, Faculty of Public Health (2010); Doctorate in Health Sciences, Orientation: Community Health from the Université Pédagogique Nationale, Doctorate in Public Health from the Université de Bangui/RCA, Licentiate in Medical Techniques, Option: Management of Health Institutions from the Institut Supérieur des Techniques Médicales de Kinshasa (ISTM-KIN), University Certified in Palliative Care and Quality of Life from the Université Catholique de Louvain (U.C.L 2010), Certified in Investigative Methods in Epidemiology and Epizootics from the School of Public Health/University of Kinshasa, Certified in Participatory Epidemiology from the School of Public Health/University of Kinshasa.

He is a member of several scientific networks and contributes to several scientific publications.

- *From 2003 to 2006, Assistant 1èr at the Institut Supérieur des Techniques Médicales de Kinshasa, Section: Gestion des Institutions de Santé ;*
- *From 2006 to 2009, Assistant 2ème mandate at the Institut Supérieur des Techniques Médicales de Kinshasa, Section: Gestion des Institutions de Santé ;*
- *From 2009 to April 2016, Chef de Travaux at the Institut Supérieur des Techniques Médicales de Kinshasa, Section: Gestion des Institutions de Santé ;*
- *From April 2016 to date, Associate Professor at the Institut Supérieur des Techniques Médicales in Kinshasa;*
- *From 2015 to the present, he is General Manager of the Institut Supérieur des Sciences de Santé de la Croix Rouge/City of Kinshasa/DRC.*

It conducts research into public health (community health), health accounting and finance, and teaches courses in epidemiology, management of health institutions, community health, health economics, project management and more.

GENERAL INTRODUCTION

Epidemiology is the study of the distribution and determinants of health and disease in populations. It forms the scientific basis of public health, and provides the tools needed to identify the causes of disease and evaluate the effectiveness of preventive and therapeutic interventions. This book explains how epidemiology enables us to move from observations to an understanding of causal relationships and the implementation of prevention strategies.

Throughout the chapters, we will address key concepts such as incidence, prevalence, association and causality. We will explore the methodologies of epidemiological studies, including cohort studies, case-control studies and randomized controlled trials. By examining the challenges of interpreting results and potential biases, this book will highlight the importance of scientific rigor in data analysis.

GENERAL OBJECTIVE

The general aim of this course is to enable readers to use epidemiological methods in the field to analyze health phenomena and their determinants in a given population with a view to control.

SPECIFIC OBJECTIVES

The specific objectives of this book are to enable readers to :

- *Determine the health status of a population in terms of the extent and distribution of health phenomena;*
- *Identify risk factors for disease or other health problems;*
- *Ensuring epidemiological surveillance in a population ;*
- *Organizing the investigation of epidemics and epizootics;*
- *Investigating and controlling epidemics and epizootics;*
- *Applying participatory epidemiology ;*
- *Integrate the one-health approach at all levels.*

CHAPTER 1: BASIC CONCEPTS IN EPIDEMIOLOGY

1.1 DEFINITION OF EPIDEMIOLOGY

Epidemiology is a science that studies the frequency and distribution of health problems or health-related phenomena in human populations, in time and space, as well as the determinants of this frequency and distribution, with the aim of controlling these problems.

The term epidemiology comes from the Greek: "Epi" (on) "demos" (population) "logos" (study of ...). Literally, epidemiology is the study of phenomena or events occurring in the population. In the past, this word referred exclusively to the "science of epidemics".

Epidemiology is concerned with the population as a whole, i.e. a group of people who are ill (what is needed) and not ill (how to prevent them from being affected).

Three fundamental elements emerge from the above definition of epidemiology:

- The frequency or extent of the health problem under study. This frequency is measured by measures of morbidity: incidence and prevalence. This is the very basis of the discipline. E.g.: find out the frequency in men and women and formulate hypotheses.

- Distribution of the health problem: a description of the health status of the population: in whom? Where? Where? i.e. person, time and place (space).

- Determinants, i.e. the risk factors that influence the occurrence of this phenomenon and its distribution in the community; the causes that influence the occurrence of health phenomena. This analysis enables us to identify the etiology of diseases.

More recently, these three elements have been joined in the field of epidemiology by the "evaluation" of healthcare initiatives.

1.2. USEFULNESS OF EPIDEMIOLOGY IN PUBLIC HEALTH

Epidemiology provides :

- Methodology for determining and monitoring the health status of the population,
- Methodology for determining priorities,
- Methodology for detecting and investigating epidemics,
- Methodology for investigating the determinants of health problems,
- Methodology for solving problems: identifying their cause(s), recommending interventions, evaluating the results of interventions.

Epidemiology involves collecting and analyzing data on the frequency and distribution of health problems, as well as on their causes. Epidemiologists must be able to provide rapid, concrete answers to community health problems, in order to inform public health decisions.

The epidemiological method enables us to put forward one or more hypotheses, verify them by means of surveys and, on the basis of the results obtained, establish new hypotheses. As the following epidemiological reasoning indicates:

Epidemiology has the following specific applications:

- Description of health problems in the population,
- Surveillance (plus control/eradication of diseases or other health problems)
- Diseases and health-related problems,
- Identifying the cause of a health problem,
- Investigating an epidemic
- Program evaluation (impact)
- Public health research

Public health is currently defined not only as a science, but also as an art whose purpose is the study, planning, implementation and evaluation of actions to improve the population's state of health. It is a set of services designed to maintain, restore and promote health-related problems.

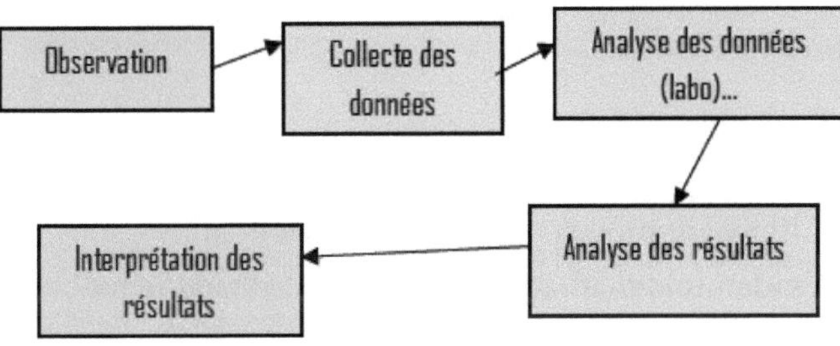

1.3 COMPARISON OF CLINICAL AND EPIDEMIOLOGICAL APPROACHES TO HEALTH PROBLEMS (TONGLET, 1995)

Table 1: Clinical versus epidemiological approach

Subject of interest	Clinical approach	Epidemiological approach
	Sick	Disease
Diagnosis	Determining the subject of clinical interest	Identification of a major group phenomenon
Search Etiological	Causes of disease onset in the subject	Causes of disease onset and spread in the population
Therapy (intervention)	Healing	Process control and eradication
Success check	Diagnosis of health improvement; monitoring the cured person	Intervention impact analysis; monitoring epidemiology of the disease

Example: Ebola virus

- Clinical approach: study the sick person
- Epidemiological approach: see the phenomena behind the virus.

Question: What advice would you give to a parent whose 5-year-old child has asthma, and who asks you whether his or her child will have asthma for the rest of his or her life?

Epidemiology is based on two assumptions:

- First, diseases do not occur and distribute randomly in populations; and
- Secondly, for every disease that strikes a population, there are triggering and preventive factors.

1.4 HISTORICAL EVOLUTION OF EPIDEMIOLOGY

Epidemiology is to some extent as old as the world itself. So, to account for the evolutionary process of epidemiology, the Public Health Agency of Canada (PHAC) has chosen to focus on the individuals, interventions and studies that have marked the discipline's past. With regard to individuals, for example, the approach is all the more justified as "many historical figures were epidemiologists who were unaware of it, long before epidemiology became a discipline, because their work bears witness to epidemiological thinking and methods" (MATUKALA 2014). Of all the precursors of epidemiology, we have selected only those who have had the greatest impact on this emerging discipline.

1.4.1 Hippocrates (460-377 BC)

Considered the father of modern medicine, Hippocrates was the first to suggest that the development of disease was linked to an individual's external and internal environment (climate, air, water, temperature, lifestyle...). Hippocrates described the symptoms and evolution of a number of diseases present in ancient Greece, such as pneumonia and mumps. His works Des épidémies I, Des épidémies II and Traité des airs, des eaux et des lieux (Treatise on Air, Water and Place) highlighted the link between disease and various natural factors, such as the seasons, geographical environment and personality. They also highlighted the importance of environmental influences on health. For Hippocrates, anyone interested in thc practice of medicine must also consider natural elements such as the wind, the season, the location of a town, the quality of the water and soil, the temperature, the lifestyle of the inhabitants, etc., since all these elements can contribute to the onset of disease. In short, diseases were caused by environmental factors both internal and external to the individual (water, temperature, climate, area, lifestyle, etc.).

1.4.2 John Graunt (1620-1674)

Graunt's work is the foundation of modern epidemiology. Indeed, while the causes of disease had been considered since Hippocrates twenty centuries earlier, it was Graunt, a London haberdasher, who first sought to measure their impact in The Nature and Political Observations Made Upon the Bills of Mortality, published in London in 1662. This was the first publication to quantify trends in births, deaths and disease. Graunt noted the imbalance in births between boys and girls, and the over-mortality of males. He coined the concept of infant mortality.

1.4.3 Thomas Sydenham (1624-1689)

Sydenham was something of a "British Hippocrates". Trained as a physician, he was known for his rigorous descriptions of diseases such as gout, malaria, measles and syphilis. The results of his descriptions made it possible to see these diseases as distinct entities. Drawing on similar work by botanists of his time, Sydenham stressed *the importance of recognizing and describing a disease*, as a first step towards understanding and ultimately preventing it.

1.4.4 Louis-René Villermé (1782-1863)

The work of French physician Villermé illustrates the growing awareness of the notion of public health during the XIXe century, a century of rapid urbanization and industrialization. Throughout the West, these major social upheavals were accompanied by a general deterioration in social conditions for workers. Villermé studied morbidity and mortality rates in Paris in 1826 and 1828, and demonstrated the close relationship between these and the living conditions of different social classes, proving in his view *the existence of a link between poverty and the onset of certain diseases.*

1.4.5 William Farr (1807-1883)

William Farr is surely one of the many putative fathers of modern epidemiology. In charge of the General Register Office and thus of medical statistics for England and Wales, Farr drew on Graunt's work to develop a system for classifying deaths (sex, age, marital status) that enabled him to confirm Villermé's conclusions about the links between health and socio-economic conditions. Because he kept a mortality register with a particular interest in the number of deaths among certain groups of individuals (miners, cast-iron workers), Farr is known as the father of vital statistics and modern monitoring. It was he who broadened the analysis of mortality and morbidity. He continued Graunt's work by setting up a classification system: sex, age, marital status...

1.4.6 John Snow (1813-1858)

Best known as Queen Victoria's anesthetist, who dared to propose chloroform anesthesia for her deliveries, Snow was also the father of "field" epidemiology. He used data collected by Farr over 40 years to test the hypothesis that cholera was transmitted by contaminated water. Indeed, Snow was astonished by the variations in the frequency of cholera in different parts of London, which had similar characteristics apart from the fact that some were supplied with water by the Southwart & Vauxhalt Company and others by the Lambeth Company. In the mid-19e century, both companies drew their water from the Thames, right in the middle of the city, but Lambeth, sensitive to criticism, moved its strainers upstream. In 1854, an outbreak of cholera gave Snow the opportunity to test the hypothesis that cholera was transmitted when a healthy person consumed water contaminated by an invisible agent found in the stools of anyone already suffering from the disease. In a district supplied by Sourtwark & Vauxhall, Snow counted a cholera incidence rate of 5%. In another neighborhood, this time supplied by Lamberth, the incidence was just 1%. In yet another district, where the two companies were in competition, the frequency was intermediate, at 2%. The transmission of cholera by drinking water, from patient to patient, was thus demonstrated. The proof of the importance of the "water supply" factor that had just been demonstrated led to the application of sanitary measures to prevent further cases of the disease.

1.4.7 Louis Pasteur (1822-1895)

Louis Pasteur inaugurated the era of medical bacteriology and immunology with his discovery that micro-organisms (microbes) were the cause of disease. **His germ theory,** enunciated in 1878, stated that the cause of infectious diseases was microscopic beings, germs (microbes), which multiplied and spread to humans through water, air, contaminated objects and direct contact between two people or between an animal and a person. This theory replaced **the miasma theory**, according to which most infectious diseases were generated and transmitted by inert (non-living) particles emanating from stagnant water, putrefaction or dirt, and were airborne (Dsrosiers and Gaumer, 2006, P. 186 cited by MATUKALA). Pasteur is remembered for his discovery of "pasteurization", the development of animal and human vaccines (against rabies, for example) and the discovery of infection mechanisms.

1.4.8 Bradford Hill (1897-1991) and Richard Doll (1912-2005)

Hill and Doll studied the relationship between smoking and lung cancer at a time when this relationship was not obvious. They found a correlation between lung cancer and smoking among British doctors. In a first study, between April 1948 and February 1952, London hospitals notified the study secretariat of 3,446 patients with cancer of the lung, stomach or large intestine. Of the eligible subjects, 2,710 were included in the study. A second "control" group of 1448 patients hospitalized for non-cancerous conditions was formed to match the lung cancer patients. After analysis, the results showed that the proportions of non-smokers and light smokers were higher among the controls and that, conversely, the proportions of very heavy smokers were greater among the cases. These differences were statically highly significant.

1.5 EPIDEMIOLOGICAL PARAMETERS: TIME, PLACE AND PERSON

To describe an epidemiological study, certain parameters, also known as variables, are used.

1.5.1 Variable definition

A variable is any character that can take on different states depending on the individual, the time or the place of observation. This term is opposed to constant.

A variable is defined as a type of observation made about an individual, time or place.

1.5.2 Variable measurement scale

These scales enable variables to be measured with a certain degree of precision. Four measurement scales have been described: nominal, ordinal, interval and ratio. In epidemiology, the first 3 scales are encountered most frequently.

a) Nominal scale: a qualitative variable

The nominal scale is the weakest of all. At this level, the values the variable can take on only indicate categories, without any notion of order or magnitude. An example of such a measurement scale is "male or female sex", which can be coded as 1 and 0 or 1 and 2, without representing any order or notion of magnitude. From a statistical point of view, it is not possible to perform mathematical operations with data from a nominal scale.

b) Ordinal scale

Although ordinal scales can also designate categories, they also have the added notion of order of magnitude. For example, groups of people receiving a certain treatment can be ordered according to a certain criterion showing the different levels (different doses) of treatment, with the high-dose group ranked ahead of the low-dose groups. Another example of a variable measured on an ordinal scale is social classes: rich, middle class, poor. Although social classes are categories, they also reveal the notion of order of magnitude. They can be ordered by trading from the poor class to the rich class. The wealthy class has more means than the middle class, and the middle class more than the poor social class.

c) Interval scale

The interval scale not only gives the notion of magnitude, but also measures the distance between categories or intervals. To be a variable measured on an interval scale, a variable must have a standardized and universally accepted measurement.

Example: temperature, height, weight, blood pressure.

d) Ratio scale

It's a scale in which different values are compared with an original value, the starting point or zero.

1.5.3 Nature of variables

Variables are not all of the same type. They are distinguished according to whether or not their values are numerical. A numerical value is called quantitative, and a non-numerical variable is called qualitative.

For example, children's weight is a numerical and therefore quantitative variable, whereas eye color is not numerical and is therefore qualitative.

a) Qualitative variable (= nominal variable = categorical variable) = non-numerical

A qualitative variable is a characteristic expressed by category, and cannot be measured in the true sense of the word. A qualitative variable is always discrete = isolated.

Examples: gender, religion, level of education, water source, health status, treatment received, blood type, conjunctival color, etc.

A quantitative variable can be converted into a qualitative variable.

Examples: age (in slices), blood pressure (in slices), number of children (in slices), blood sugar (in slices).

Application: the results of observing a qualitative variable are expressed by category.

b) Quantitative variable (= numerical variable)

A quantitative variable is one that can actually be measured; it is expressed by numerical values. The variable may be discrete or continuous.

- **Discrete variable (= isolated)**

It can only take on distinct and separate (discontinuous) numerical values. Between the values it can take on, there is no possibility of finding other values. These variables are expressed as integers. The value of an isolated variable cannot be measured; it is obtained by enumeration.

Example: number of children per family, parity, episodes of diarrhea.

- **Continuous variable (= not isolated)**

The values of this type of variable can be expressed as real numbers, i.e. numbers with decimal digits. Between the values it can assume, there is a continuous (uninterrupted) series of numerical values.

Example: Ages, blood pressure, blood sugar, weight, height, Hb level.

Application: results of observations made on a quantitative variable are expressed as mean, minimum/maximum, standard deviation, etc.

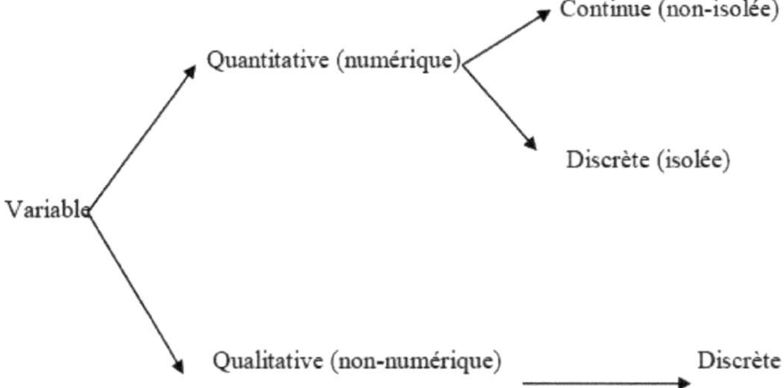

1.5.4 Variable types

The variables used in clinical and epidemiological studies can be grouped according to the three aspects that characterize exposure or disease: person variables, place variables and time variables.

1.5.4.1 People variables

They refer to anatomical, physiological, social or cultural attributes,

- WHO is affected?
- Expressed as: age, gender, marital status, ethnicity, religion, education level, socio-economic level, degree of exposure to suspected risk factors (e.g. cigarettes, radioactivity, meals, etc.), behavior, attitude, practice, household size, heredity......
- Expressed by: table, graph.

Person variables answer the question "WHO?

1.5.4.2 Location variables

These variables take into account the geographical distribution of the frequency of exposure factors and diseases.

- WHERE are the cases?
- Expressed in: planet, continent, country, province, district, territory, village, household
- Expressed by map, often in relation to a landmark (river, mountains, suspected source of the problem, etc.).

Environmental variables answer the question "Where?

1.5.4.3 Time variables

Time variables are used to characterize how an exposure or disease varies over time.

- WHEN did the cases appear?
- Expressed in: epoch, century, decade, year, month, week, day, hour, minute, observation time
- Expressed by: graph (epidemiological curve), table.

Time variables are used to answer the question "WHEN".

1.5.5 Relationship between variables

The study of relationships between various variables enables them to be divided into independent and dependent variables.

- In theory, an independent variable is one whose evolution is not affected by other variables. In practice, it is a potentially explanatory variable, a potentially causal factor, whose effect we are seeking to evaluate. If, for example, we want to study the relationship between the frequency of respiratory illnesses and air pollution, air pollution will be considered an independent variable.
- One dependent variable varies according to another. In practice, when we use the cause-effect model, we consider that the dependent variable is the one that enables us to

measure the effect under study. In the example above, the dependent variable is the frequency of respiratory illnesses.

Table 2: Variables in an "exposure-disease" contingency table

VARIABLE INDEPENDENT = Exposure or Cause	DEPENDENT VARIABLE = Disease or Effect		
	Patients	No - sick	
Presentations	A	B	a + b
Non-exposed	C	D	c + d
	a + c	b + d	a + b + c + d

Question: how does epidemiology go about establishing the relationship between lung cancer in a society where every adult smokes at least 20 cigarettes a day?

1.5.6 Epidemics, endemics and pandemics

Table 3: Differences between epidemics, endemics and pandemics

	Number of cases	emps	Spaces (Location)
Epidemic	High	Limited	imited
Endemic	High	Unlimited	Limited
Pandemic	High	Limited	Unlimited

1.5.6.1 Epidemics

An epidemic is a sudden development and rapid spread of a communicable or non-communicable disease that simultaneously affects a large number of individuals over a limited period of time, in a given territory or community. It is manifested by the unusual appearance of a large number of cases where the disease does not exist, or by a considerable increase in the number of cases when the disease is endemic in the region or population concerned. It is the occurrence within a population of a significantly higher-than-usual number of cases of a given disease (often ≥10%, except for rare diseases).

Question: - When can an epidemic be declared?

- can malaria become an epidemic? Justify your answer.

An epidemic is a mass phenomenon, limited in time and space.

Example: Ebola in Kikwit, Monkeypox in Sankuru.

In animals, the same phenomenon is called an "epizootic".

There's a difference between an epidemic and an outbreak. An outbreak is an epidemic in a small population.

1.5.6.2 Endemic

An endemic is the habitual presence, in a region or population, of a disease that occurs constantly or periodically. It is the constant presence of a disease (habitual prevalence) at an equal frequency over a long period of time. Endemic differs from epidemic in that the former is unlimited in time but limited in space, whereas the latter is limited in time and space. It is the constant (permanent) presence of a disease (habitual prevalence) at a legal level of frequency over a long period of time.

It's a mass phenomenon, unlimited and limited in space.

Unlimited time = many cases of disease over several successive generations.

Example: - Malaria in the DRC

-Trypanosomiasis in the DRC

With animals, we talk about "Enzootie".

1.5.6.3 Pandemic

A pandemic is the appearance of a series of cases limited in time but not in space. Unlimited space is represented by the case where the disease spreads throughout the entire population, or several continents and their respective populations are affected. This is the distribution of a disease on a global scale, i.e. across borders.

Examples: - Influenza

- HIV

For animals, this is called "Panzootie".

1.6 BASIC MODEL OF EPIMIOLOGICAL REASONING

The "Pasteurian" or biomedical model that underpins the teaching of medicine establishes a hypothetical causal relationship between an agent and a host. If the interaction is balanced, we are dealing with a state of "health". If, on the other hand, the interaction is out of balance, we're in a state of disease.

In clinical practice, the physician takes a history to determine the causal agent of a pathology (i.e., to diagnose a disease by asking questions).

The epidemiological model takes an additional element into account: the environment (physical, social and biological). In other words, the causal agent must find a suitable terrain in which to develop, so that the host is affected. It is therefore an "ecological" model, which sees health as a state of equilibrium between three factors (the triad or epidemiological triangle):

- The individual (host): this comprises a set of factors intrinsic to an individual that affect his or her exposure, sensitivity or reaction to a causal agent (age, lifestyle, socioeconomic status, etc.). Host susceptibility depends on a number of factors: genetic, nutritional, etc.
- The causal agent: this may be infectious or a non-infectious risk factor (e.g. virus, bacteria, chemical substance, etc.).
- The environment: this encompasses the factors influencing the agent and the possibility of exposure. These include physical factors (e.g. climate), biological factors (e.g. insects) and socio-economic factors (e.g. access to health services).

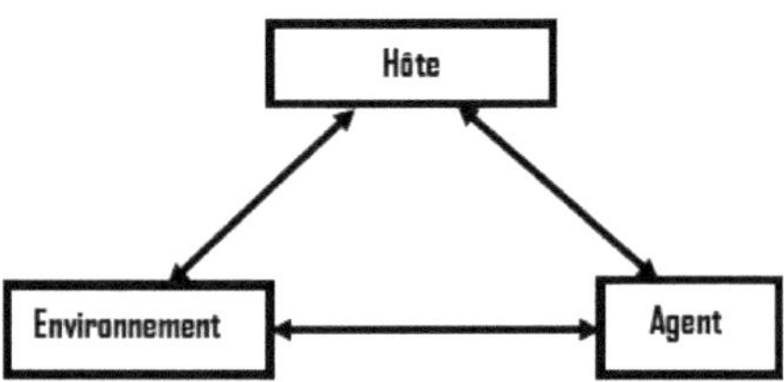

1.7. EPIDEMIOLOGICAL DATA SOURCES

There are two types of epidemiological data.

- Data collected on an ongoing basis, i.e. "routine" data and epidemiological surveillance data.
- Data deliberately collected as part of epidemiological surveys.

These two sources of data complement each other, since, for example, an epidemiological survey can be organized to make better use of "routine" data, while basic demographic data are indispensable for planning the sampling of an observational study.

1.7.1 Data collected on a permanent basis

1.7.1.1 Vital statistics

They include systematically collected facts that are represented in digital form. They include life events such as live births, marriages, divorces and adoptions.

Examples of civil status documents.

- Live births

They are usually recorded on a document called a "birth certificate". This document is of the utmost importance. A certificate without a birth certificate does not legally exist. This document provides information on the birth, sex, place, date and, generally, the circumstances surrounding the birth.

- Deaths

The concept of death is reported on a certificate called a death certificate. This certificate provides information on gender, cause of death, illnesses or events that led to death, and the date of death.

1.7.1.2 Censuses

They consist in counting the population over a given period of time. Censuses provide information on the size of the population at any given time. They provide the denominator for calculating various rates used in epidemiology.

1.7.1.3. Health statistics

These statistics come from institutions offering both curative and promotional services. They include :

a) Hospital statistics

They provide information on morbidity and mortality in the population. Unfortunately, these data are rarely representative of the population, since not all patients go to hospital. Medical records are difficult to use.

b) Statistics from insurers

They concern subscribers only. So they don't cover the whole population. On the other hand, many organizations are more concerned with the details of drugs than with diagnoses.

c) Statistics from compulsory disease declarations

Unfortunately, few institutions systematically report on these diseases. We often resort to data recorded on specific populations (= captive populations) such as schools or the army.

1.7.1.4 The police or gendarmerie

These institutions have data on road accidents and other events.

1.7.1.5 Schools and other training institutions

They provide data for school medical services, for example.

1.7.2 Epidemiological surveys

These surveys are organized to produce the information needed to achieve specific objectives: measuring the extent of a problem, etiological research, evaluating an intervention, etc.

1.8 THE HEALTH CONCEPT

The WHO has proposed the following definition of health: "Health is a state of complete physical, mental and social well-being and not merely the absence of disease or infirmity.

Despite the criticism it has received for the difficulties of defining and measuring "complete well-being", this definition nevertheless allows us to approach the question of health in three distinct and complementary ways:

- Perceptual approach, which defines health as a subjective perception of well-being;
- A functional approach that describes health as the ability to function well in a particular physical, psychological and social environment;
- Adaptive approach, using the concept of the individual's adaptation to its environment

It should be noted, however, that it is difficult to give a simple definition of health, because health is multifactorial. On the other hand, it is easy to define illness and a health problem.

- Disease is an abnormal biological process, often explicable and classifiable according to its causes and mechanisms.
- A health problem is defined as actual or potential suffering resulting from a process that disrupts the state of health and causes a state of individual or collective "ill-being".

1.9 HEALTH DETERMINANTS

As mentioned above, the main determinants of psycho-socio-somatic health are related to the environment, individual behaviour, the human being (in particular heredity = intrinsic factors) and the factors governing health provision (health services). There is thus an interaction between the population, the behavior of the population, the environment and the health services, one controlling the other and one influencing the other.

Key health determinants

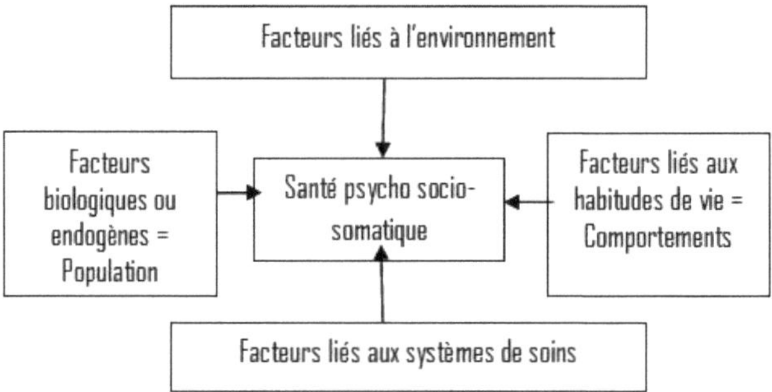

This means that the organization of health services alone cannot guarantee psycho-socio-somatic health.

CHAPTER 2: STATISTICAL ASSOCIATION AND THE NOTION OF CAUSALITY

The aim of this chapter is twofold: firstly, to present how to assess a valid statistical association between an exposure and a disease; secondly, to describe the notion of causality by unveiling some causal models in epidemiology. This description will not fail to underline the dynamic nature of the causes of health and disease, as well as the mechanisms for preventing health problems within a population.

2.1 ASSESSING THE VALIDITY OF A STATISTICAL ASSOCIATION

The term association refers to a statistical relationship between two variables, i.e. the extent to which the frequency of a disease or health condition in subjects with a specific exposure differs, plus or minus, from the frequency of that disease in non-exposed subjects (Matukala op.cit). While the results of an epidemiological study may be the actual consequence of an exposure on the development of a disease, they may also reflect factors other than the exposure concerned. This is why, in the presence of a statistical association, we must always ask questions before concluding that it is valid. There are in fact two types of validity to be verified: *external validity*, where the researcher ensures that the results of his study can be generalized to other populations, and *internal validity,* where he ensures that chance, selection or information bias, and confusion due to certain variables do not explain the results obtained.

Let's take a closer look at these last three elements.

2.1.1 The role of chance

Indeed, whenever a population sample is examined, it is possible that the association observed between an exposure and a disease is due to chance, a situation known as random error. Sample size is one of the main factors influencing the proportion of chance in study results.

2.1.2 The role of bias

The presence of bias is one of the explanations for an observable statistical association between an exposure and a disease. A bias is a systematic error introduced during the design or execution of a study. Biases may therefore be present in the way individuals are selected, in the way information is obtained or in the way it is presented. This is particularly the case when the method of selecting individuals differs according to whether they are cases or controls, and this difference is related to their exposure status. Similarly, if methods for collecting, analyzing or interpreting information differ between groups in the same study, there is a risk of observing a relationship when it does not actually exist.

There are two main types of bias: selection bias and information bias. Selection bias occurs when participants in a study are not selected on the basis of comparable criteria. Information bias, on the other hand, occurs when non-comparable information or information of different quality is obtained from study participants.

2.1.3 The role of confusion

Confounding represents a third possible explanation for an observed statistical association, as it may be the consequence of other fundamental differences between groups that were not measured. In other words, the observed statistical association may result from a mixture of effects between the exposure, the disease and a third factor associated with the exposure and acting independently on the risk of developing the disease. This phenomenon is called confounding, and the external factor just mentioned is the confounding variable.

2.2 ESTABLISHING A CAUSE-AND-EFFECT RELATIONSHIP

When chance, bias and confounding are ruled out in a study, it becomes correct, on the basis of the study data, to conclude that there is a valid statistical association between exposure and disease (Hennekens et al, 1998). A valid statistical association can be a causal or cause-and-effect relationship, and the main aim of epidemiology is to verify whether this is the case. To achieve this, it is necessary to base judgment on certain criteria.

2.3 BRADFORD HILL'S CAUSALITY CRITERIA

These criteria give aspects to consider when distinguishing between causal and non-causal associations. These criteria are :

1. Strength of association - According to this criterion, the stronger the association between an outcome and an exposure, the more likely it is that the association is causal. The strength of the association is defined by the magnitude of the risk, itself measured by appropriate statistics.
2. Consistency of association - Consistency of association is said to exist if the association is consistently observed despite studies being carried out in different contexts using different methods. In such circumstances, it is unlikely that all studies will make the same mistake. *To arrive at the same result when you do the same analyses, i.e. each time the association is calculated in the same context, it must establish the association as it has already been done*.

3. Specificity - Specificity is established when a single presumed cause produces a specific effect. Hill warns, however, against attributing undue importance to this criterion. Indeed, when dealing with multifactorial diseases, this criterion is of very limited use, and may even prove invalid. There is only one cause to explain a disease A→B
4. Chronological sequence - It's vital that the exposure precedes the result in time. This criterion is absolutely essential. The cause (exposure) must precede the consequence (disease).
5. Biological gradient (dose-response relationship) - This criterion means that an increased level of exposure, in quantity or duration, corresponds to an increased risk of disease. The more you are exposed, the more you develop the disease.
   EX: the more you smoke, the more cancer you develop.
6. Biological plausibility - The association must conform to what pathological mechanisms predict. *In other words, what science has established.* Whether this criterion is met depends on the degree of biological knowledge attained in the field in question.
   Alcohol →accident} → that explains it
   Tobacco →cancer}
   Drink alcohol → pleasure, without any other mechanism.
7. Consistency (compatibility): The association must be comparable with existing theory and knowledge.
8. Experimental evidence: This criterion is met if there is evidence that the state of health or disease can be modified by an appropriate experimental regimen. This criterion therefore refers to proof obtained by eliminating a harmful exposure as part of an intervention or prevention program.

It must be scientifically demonstrated that if you remove the cause, the consequence will no longer exist.
Alcohol → cancer (no alcohol,

9. Analogy — For Hill, experience of one situation can lead to the consideration of analogous results for similar exposures to other diseases.

2.4 DISEASE TRANSMISSION MODES

According to Gordis (2004), disease transmission can be direct or indirect. Direct transmission occurs when one factor causes the disease directly, without passing through an intermediary factor. On the other hand, indirect transmission occurs when a factor causes the disease through other factors in one or more intermediate stages. Indirect transmission can be either horizontal or vertical. Horizontal transmission occurs indirectly via a common vehicle (single, multiple or continuous exposure), through direct person-to-person contact or via a vector. Vertical transmission occurs from mother to child during pregnancy.

Table 4: Disease transmission modes

Modes of disease transmission (Gordis, 2014)	
Direct (cross-transmission)	**Indirect**
Direct person-to-person contact	A. Horizontal transmission 1. Shared vehicle : a) Single exposure (1 single factor) b) Multiple exposure (several factors) c)Continuous exposure (smokers) Ex: Consumption of contaminated food or water responsible for gastroenteritis. 2. Vector B. Vertical transmission (from mother to child during pregnancy).

a. Direct or cross-transmission: when one factor directly causes the disease without passing through an intermediary factor.

   E.g.: human-to-human transmission of tuberculosis by air.

b. Indirect transmission: when a factor causes the disease through other factors in one or more intermediate stages.

CHAPTER 3: PREVENTION AND SCREENING

3.1 PREVENTION

Prevention is the set of measures aimed at avoiding the development of diseases or their consequences.

3.1.1 Natural history of the disease :

This is the natural evolution of the disease in a subject from onset to resolution, in the absence of any intervention.

It is the natural history of the disease that largely determines the possibilities for prevention. The model of this natural history can be represented as a set of causal hypotheses linking together four successive stages (Rotham, 1981; Kleinbaum et al, 1982).

1. The stage of initiation of the etiological process (sensitivity stage), which is reached as soon as the subject is exposed to the effect of one or more risk factors (e.g. the effects of tobacco, alcohol, a pollutant, another disease, the expression of an infectious risk, etc.). At this stage, only the risk factors are present.
2. The stage of initiation of the pathological process or pre-clinical or pre-symptomatic stage, which is reached when pre-symptomatic physiological alterations have occurred (e.g. development of cervical cancer in situ, insidious installation of atherosclerosis lesions, development of interstitial pulmonary fibrosis, acquisition of an infectious state without clinical manifestations, etc.) which will evolve towards disappearance, stabilization or aggravation and irreversibility. The etiological agent is present in the body and causes pathological changes, but without producing perceptible signs or symptoms.

3. The disease manifestation or symptomatic stage, which is reached when the disease has become symptomatic. This is the stage at which the signs or symptoms of the disease appear in the subject.
4. The disease resolution or late clinical stage, which is reached at the end of the natural history of the disease, when it has progressed to cure (spontaneous or not), cure with residual abnormality, chronicity or death.

The process of moving from one of these states to another can be broken down into three phases:

1. The induction phase, during which the exposed subject experiences pre-symptomatic physiological changes that may be irreversible;
2. The promotion phase, during which the subject moves from the pre-clinical stage to the clinical stage of the disease by becoming a symptomatic patient;
3. The disease expression phase, during which the disease progresses until its final outcome.

The phases of disease induction and promotion together form what is known as the disease latency phase, i.e. the time interval between the moment when the first disease-causing factor is implemented and the moment when the disease is detected. This phase is of fundamental interest to ethological research (the study of the causes of disease).

The expression phase of the disease is complementary to the latency phase, and corresponds to what is most often referred to as the duration of the disease. This phase is the main focus of clinical research (study of the effects and impact of medical care).

The combination of latency and duration defines the chronic nature of a disease. A disease can be described as chronic either because its natural history is long (latency + duration), or because its clinical manifestations are of long duration. The concept of chronicity is therefore dimensional:

1. Short latency, short duration (e.g. flu)
2. Short latency, long duration (e.g. syphilis)
3. Long latency, short duration (e.g. pancreatic cancer)
4. Long latency, long duration (e.g. hypertension)

These same observations can, however, be used in an entirely different way for action. Each of the three phases in the natural history of the disease corresponds to an opportunity for intervention:

1. The disease-induction phase is followed by the primary prevention phase, during which it is possible to prevent exposure to a risk factor or limit its consequences (e.g. changes in dietary habits or lifestyle, vaccination, control of food nuisances, etc.), i.e. to try to prevent the onset of disease (reduce the incidence of disease). Health protection through personal and community efforts.
2. The phase of disease promotion is followed by the phase of secondary prevention, during which it is possible to halt the evolution of the pathogenic process (e.g., suggesting that a coronary smoker stop smoking, removing a pre-clinical cancer lesion, providing drug-based blood pressure control for a hypertensive patient, etc.), i.e., to try to reduce the proportion of disease in the population (reduce the prevalence of disease);
3. The expression phase of the disease is followed by the tertiary prevention phase, during which attempts are made to limit the consequences of a disease that has become

symptomatic, i.e. to administer curative care to patients. Actions are aimed at reducing the serious consequences of the disease or health problem. These serious consequences may be deficiencies, incapacities or handicaps.

These three levels of prevention are of great importance in public health. Medicine cannot be reduced to curative care. Health professionals, like other players in the health field (the population, political leaders, etc.), have to make choices from among a range of possible actions.

- Impairment: encompasses anything that disrupts the normal functioning (physical, mental and social) of the individual.
- Disability: is a functional limitation or restriction of activity resulting from an impairment.
- Disability: is an exclusion from social roles or places as a result of an impairment or incapacity.

Conceptual model of the natural history of the disease, according to Kleinbaum et al.

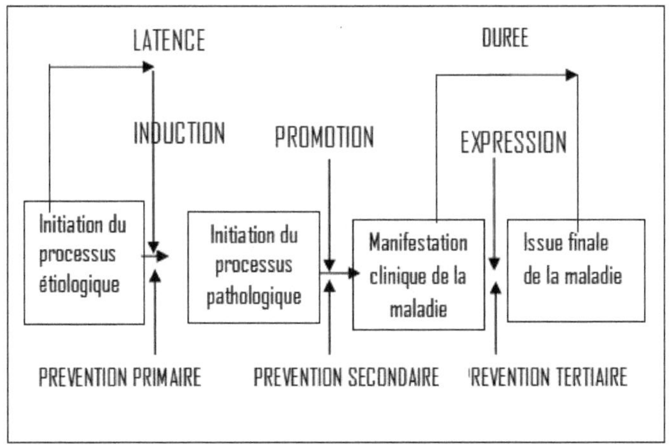

3.1.2 Prevention level

It is currently accepted that there are four levels of prevention.

These four levels correspond to the different phases in the evolution of a disease.

1. Prevention is key;
2. Primary prevention ;
3. Secondary prevention ;
4. Tertiary prevention

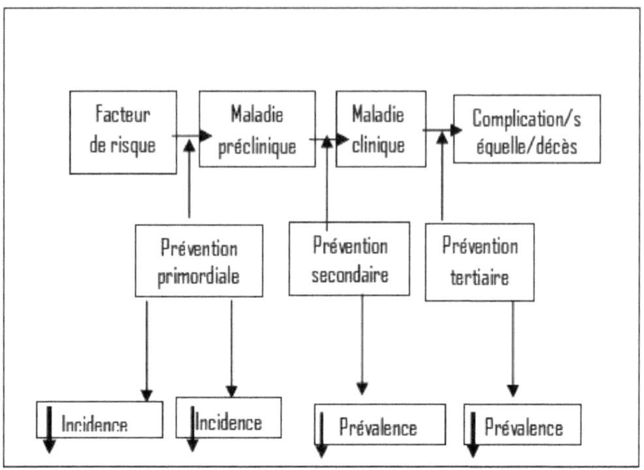

3.1.2.1 Primary prevention

Prevention is primarily aimed at factors that promote the action of the disease's specific etiological factors.

The aim of primary prevention is to prevent the adoption and maintenance of social, economic and cultural attitudes and lifestyles that predispose to a high risk of disease.

Prevention will be all the more effective if the public authorities support it, notably by putting in place regulations and/or policies to back it up.

Let's take an example:

To combat iodine deficiency, the most important preventive measure is to introduce import regulations for cooking salt, educate the population to consume only iodized salt, and encourage retailers to import only iodized salt. The key to prevention is therefore to combat the onset of risk factors.

3.1.2.2 Primary prevention

Action in the disease induction phase, with the aim of reducing the frequency of occurrence (incidence) by acting on the causes and risk factors.

Examples: individual and community hygiene measures, vaccination.

Primary prevention takes place at the stage of host susceptibility. In fact, the host susceptibility stage is the ideal time to implement primary prevention, since at this stage the disease has not yet begun, but all the risk factors are present. For example, in the case of measles, a child has recently arrived in a measles-endemic area, has not been vaccinated against measles, and is twelve months old, so has almost already exhausted the protective antibodies inherited from his mother. As a result, this child is likely to contract measles. Acting now will counteract the effect of these risk factors.

Primary prevention is a set of measures that affect risk factors so that they do not affect the host, with the aim of preventing the outbreak of the disease. It intervenes in disease-free individuals before they fall ill. These measures could be general health promotion actions, such as the promotion of good nutrition or hygiene at home, at work, and so on. Health education thus has its place in primary prevention. Primary prevention is aimed at preventing the onset of disease, and thus at reducing its incidence.

3.1.2.3 Secondary prevention

Action in the disease promotion phase, aimed at preventing the disease from progressing from the pre-clinical to the clinical stage.

Examples: -Early detection and treatment of diseases.

Secondary prevention has two aims: to cure disease and to mitigate its most serious effects through early diagnosis and treatment. Secondary prevention contributes to reducing prevalence.

In the asymptomatic stage, even if the disease has not yet manifested itself, pathogenic changes are gaining ground on the individual. In terms of disease progression, we're talking about the incubation period. The incubation period is the time interval between the entry of the infectious agent and the onset of the disease. It should be noted that the incubation period, a term reserved for infectious diseases, corresponds to the latency period for non-infectious diseases. Here, the mild form of the disease is often asymptomatic. Secondary prevention focuses on the asymptomatic stage of the disease. It reduces the duration of the disease's evolution. For example, educating the adult population to have their blood pressure checked regularly aims to detect hypertension at the stage when it is still benign, so that treatment can prevent the disease from progressing to the advanced stage. The aim of secondary prevention is therefore to reduce the prevalence of the disease.

3.1.2.4 Tertiary prevention

Action in the expression phase of the disease. This means preventing deterioration, complications and relapses. This level of prevention is that of curative medicine.

Tertiary prevention aims to avoid complications, reduce the impact of disability, rehabilitate the function of a limb or organ affected by sequelae, or prevent the patient's death. It takes place once the disease has manifested itself and run its course long enough to cause residual damage. Tertiary prevention measures include specific treatment of the disease and its complications, or physiotherapy to restore limb function, or the fitting of a prosthesis to improve the hearing of a hearing-impaired person who has suffered from poorly treated otitis. Physiotherapy for a hemiplegic who has suffered a stroke can help reintegrate him/her into daily social life.

Tertiary prevention also focuses on social and professional reintegration after the disease. It reduces the frequency of disability and recurrence.

It's important to note that primary prevention has made the greatest contribution to the health and well-being of the entire population.

For secondary and tertiary prevention, early diagnosis using valid, rapid tests that can be applied on a large scale is essential.

3.2. MASS SCREENING FOR DISEASE DETECTION

Clearly, the ideal approach to disease control is primary prevention, i.e. preventing the disease in the first place. When primary prevention is not possible, the priority becomes early detection and treatment. For this, there are2 possibilities: screening at the very first signs of disease, or even earlier screening of asymptomatic people.

Screening from the earliest signs still depends on doctors and the public themselves to recognize and respond early to the onset of these signs. This chapter focuses on the early detection of asymptomatic, apparently healthy people, in order to intervene as early as possible in the course of the disease.

3.2.1 Definition

Mass screening is the process of diagnosing previously undetected diseases or deficiencies, using tests that can be applied rapidly and on a large scale.

This is the application of tests or examinations to an apparently healthy population or individuals, with the aim of distinguishing subjects who are likely to be free of a given disease from subjects with the previously undetected disease, in order to institute further examinations, preventive measures or treatment.

For recognized by the application of tests, examinations or other procedures that are quickly usable and enable us to distinguish between people who probably have the disease (or condition) and those who probably do not. A screening test is not necessarily a diagnosis. Those suspected positive (by the test) should be sent to their doctor for definitive diagnosis and treatment (if necessary). (OKITOLONDA 2015).

3.2.2. Purpose

The aim of screening is to determine who has the problem in the population, usually through a widely available test.

Examples: glycemia (diabetes), blood pressure (hypertension), proteinuria (eclampsia), serological test (HIV), Papa Nicolau smear (cervical cancer).

Mass screening has several applications:

1. In an epidemiological study: determining prevalence or progression

Natural disease ;

2. Prevention of contagion and protection of public health (e.g. tuberculosis) ;

3. Screening at the individual level, for better treatment.

3.2.3 Characteristics of a screening test

The important characteristics of a mass screening test are :

- Validity (sensitivity, specificity),
- Reliability (reproducibility),
- Yield,
- Speed,
- Low cost,
- Innocuousness,
- Feasibility by technicians (not necessarily by specialists).

Reliability

A reliable test must give the same result each time it is applied to the same individual under the same conditions. There are two sources of result variability: inter-individual (between 2 people interpreting the test) and intra-individual (variability of several test readers by the same individual). Thus, there are two factors that influence test reliability:

- Variability inherent in the method itself ;
- Variability due to the observer (between observers or between observations from the same observer).

Normally, these errors can be controlled by: standardization of procedures and equipment, proper training of observers, periodic supervision of their work, and/or the use of 2 (or more) observers who interpret results independently.

It should be noted that if the variability of a test is excessive, the usefulness of the test is compromised.

Performance

The yield of a test refers to the number of previously unrecognized cases diagnosed by screening and put on treatment.

The factors that influence performance are :

1. Disease incidence ;

2. Prevalence of the disease in its pre-clinical (asymptomatic) phase ;

3. The population targeted by the screening program (higher yield in higher-risk individuals, e.g. screening for diabetes in people >40 years of age, the obese, or those with a family history of diabetes). One of the problems with screening is that most cases are often found among people who apparently have no risk factors.

Once the program's yield begins to decline, it should be reviewed to assess whether it is still useful, or whether the target population cannot be redefined. Overall yield can be increased if several tests (for several diseases) are administered at the same visit (e.g., breast cancer, cervical cancer, hypertension, glaucoma).

3.2.4 Requirements for screening

- Screening should only be recommended if an intervention can be carried out. This intervention will have an impact on the individual or the population (e.g. diabetes, hypertension, proteinuria - correct treatment; HIV-positive - advice to contacts to avoid transmission);

- Screening is not appropriate if no intervention is available to prolong the life of the individual or to reduce the impact on the population (e.g. if cervical cancer is not curable, there would be no point in early screening, as the patient would suffer unnecessarily).
- Screening can be mass (campaign). In this case, the disease must be serious (severity +++, prevalence ↑). Example: Trypanosomiasis in an endemic region. The concept of screening implicitly assumes that, carried out early, before the onset of symptoms, the prognosis will be improved, as treatment instituted before the onset of obvious clinical manifestations will be more effective than late treatment.
- Screening can also be individual or targeted at high-risk individuals.

Example: People working with lead or asbestos.

For example, in males over the age of 50, have a prostate exam.

- The success of a screening program depends very much on the participation of the target population. A screening program cannot help improve the health of the population if it does not participate in screening and treatment. There are 4 factors that influence population participation:
    - The population must sense the threat of the disease (the individual must be aware of the disease);
    - People need to take the disease seriously;
    - The individual must feel vulnerable to the disease (if he doesn't feel at risk, he probably won't take part in the program);
    - He needs to believe that screening can be of use to him.

Population participation includes acceptance of the test, cooperation in the interview and compliance with further diagnosis or treatment if necessary. The program also requires medical staff to take necessary action in response to positive test results;

If the disease in question is seen as a serious, personal threat, and if screening is seen as an opportunity to avert that threat, the population's participation is better assured; if not, participation may be compromised.

3.2.5 Factors to consider when setting up a screening program

1. The condition (or disease) must be a significant health problem. Indeed, given the investment of resources, screening should only be undertaken when there is hope of significantly reducing the rate of disability or mortality;

2. There must be an acceptable treatment for the cases (... do not undertake screening if there is no treatment);

3. Facilities for definitive diagnosis and treatment must be available;

4. A valid test or examination is required;

5. It must have a "latent" or preclinical phase (even early signs), *because the disease must be detected early in the asymptomatic phase in order to detect damage and manage it for treatment*;

6. The test must be acceptable to the entire population;

7. The natural progression of the disease, its development from the "latent" phase to the disease phase, must be sufficiently well understood. *Because when we are at the etiological initiation stage, we need to know the mechanism, the cause of transmission of the disease*;

8. A case management program must be in place;

9. The cost of screening (including definitive diagnosis and possible treatment) must be compared with the cost of subsequent treatment of an already advanced case (... Cost-effectiveness, cost-benefit analysis), *i.e. what is the ratio between the cost of screening and the cost of* treatment?

10. The program must be a continuous process for identifying cases, and not "a one-off (case-by-case), cross-cutting (permanent) exercise".

3.3 VALIDITY AND USEFULNESS OF A SCREENING TEST

3.3.1 The informative value of observation data

Table 5: Relationship between a test result and the presence of a disease

Test	**Disease**	
	Present	Absent
Positive	A True positive	B False positive
Negative	C False negative	D True negative

3.3.2 Intrinsic validity of a test in relation to a reference method

- Sensitivity
- Specific

The informative value of a test is always relative to a reference method against which all other approaches must be compared (the "gold standard", which provides the information closest to reality, according to our current state of knowledge).

The ***intrinsic*** validity of a test depends on its ability to provide a positive result in patients who are ill and a negative result in those who are not, or, more precisely, to recognize patients previously identified as ill and not ill on the basis of a reference test. The parameters that measure a test's intrinsic value are its sensitivity and specificity.

A test's ***sensitivity*** is its ability to give a positive result when the disease is present. In the language of probability, sensitivity measures the conditional probability of the test being positive when the disease is present. Sensitivity is estimated by the proportion of positive results among patients, i.e. the ratio of true positives to total patients. This proportion is expressed as follows:

Se = total true positives/total patients

ou

a/ (a+c)

Specificity is the probability that a test will give a negative result in non-diseased people. It refers to a test's ability to detect non-diseased individuals, or to exclude diseased subjects. It is therefore the proportion of subjects with a negative test among non-diseased subjects. This proportion is obtained by the following formula:

Sp = total true negatives/total non-diseased

Ou

d/(b+d)

3.3.3 The predictive validity or usefulness of a test in the context of observation

- **VPP**

- **VPN**

We have seen that, in order to measure sensitivity and specificity, it is necessary to first determine the patient's actual condition by means of a reference test. However, in clinical practice or when collecting epidemiological observations, the investigator obviously does not know this actual state. He seeks to know it by performing the test, or rather he seeks to estimate the probability of the disease on the basis of the test results.

The predictive validity of a test depends on its ability to provide a positive or negative result that corresponds to a high probability of the presence or absence of the disease. The indices that measure the predictive validity of a test are the positive predictive value of a positive test and the negative predictive value of a negative test.

The positive predictive value of a positive test measures the conditional probability that the disease will be present when the test is positive. It is the a posteriori probability of the presence of a disease after a positive test. The positive predictive value of a positive test is estimated by the proportion of patients among test-positive subjects, i.e. the ratio of true positives to total positives.

The negative predictive value of a negative test measures the conditional probability that the disease is absent when the test is negative. It is the a posteriori probability of absence of a disease after a negative test. The negative predictive value of a negative test is estimated by the proportion of non-diseased subjects among those negative to the test. In other words, the ratio of true negatives to total negatives.

Table 6: BASIC TEST EVALUATION PLAN

TEST STUDY	REFERENCE TEST		TOTAL
	Patients	Sains	
Positive result	VP	FP	VP+FP
Negative result	FN	VN	FN+VN
Total	VP+FN	FP+VN	VP+FP+FN+ VN

- VP: really positive results (positive results in sick subjects)
- FP: false-positive results (positive results in healthy subjects)
- FN: false-negative results (negative results in sick subjects)
- VN: truly negative results (negative results in healthy subjects)

Several information can be obtained on the value of the test studied:

Sensitivity = $\frac{VP}{VP+FN} x\ 100$

Specificity = $\frac{VN}{VN+FP} x\ 100$

Predictive value of a positive result = 1 $\frac{VP}{VP+FP} x\ 100$

Predictive value of negative result = 1 $\frac{VN}{VN+FN} x\ 100$

Overall test value = $\frac{VP+VN}{VP+FP+FN+VN} x\ 100$

REFERENCE TEST

Table 7: GOLD STANDARD / ETALON /VERITE

	Disease	No disease	
Disease	A	B	a+b
No disease	C	D	c+d
Total	a+c	b+d	n

- **a + c**: True patients (**a** = true positive by test, **c** = false negative by test)
- **b + d:** True non-patients (**b** = false positive by text, **d** = true negative by test)
- **a + b:** Total positive by test (**a** = vari positive, **b** = false positive)
- **c + d:** Total negative by test (**c** = false negative, **d** = true negative)

Ideal is that the b and c cells contain no subjects; in other words, that the test perfectly identifies true positives and true negatives.

Practical interpretation of the table

- Sensitivity: how many true positives are detected by the test (a/a+c)
- Specificity: How many true negatives are identified as negative by the test? (d/b+d)
- Positive predictive value (PPV): What is the probability that someone identified as positive by the test will be positive (a/a+b)?
- Negative predictive value: What is the probability that someone identified as negative by the test will actually be negative? (d/c+d)
- Overall test efficiency (value): What is the percentage of test subjects correctly classified as positive or negative? (a+d/n)

3.3.4. Bayes' theorem

The predictive validity of a test is highly dependent on the context in which it is performed.

The positive or negative predictive value of a test is the result of the interaction between the frequency of the disease in the population studied, the sensitivity of the test and its specificity. This can easily be demonstrated by applying the rules of probability calculus.

One of these rules, called Bayes' theorem, calculates the positive predictive value and the negative predictive value as follows:

$$VPP = \frac{Prévalence\ x\ Se}{(\text{Prévalence x Se}) + (1 - \text{Prévalence})\ \text{x}\ (1 - \text{Sp})}$$

$$VPN = \frac{(1 - \text{Prévalence})\text{x Sp}}{(1 - \text{prévalence})\ \text{x Sp} + (\text{prévalence})\text{x}\ (1 - \text{Se})}$$

CHAPTER 4: EPIDEMIOLOGICAL STUDIES

4.1 INTRODUCTION

From mortality and morbidity studies carried out in a community, the epidemiologist can observe a statistical association between a population characteristic and the occurrence of a disease. This association may, however, be spurious. In a 2ème second step, the epidemiologist can try to confirm this association by conducting epidemiological studies with the intention of determining whether the association is present in the group of individuals with the characteristic in question and absent in the group of individuals without said characteristic.

Figure Types of epidemiological studies (PHAC, 2005)

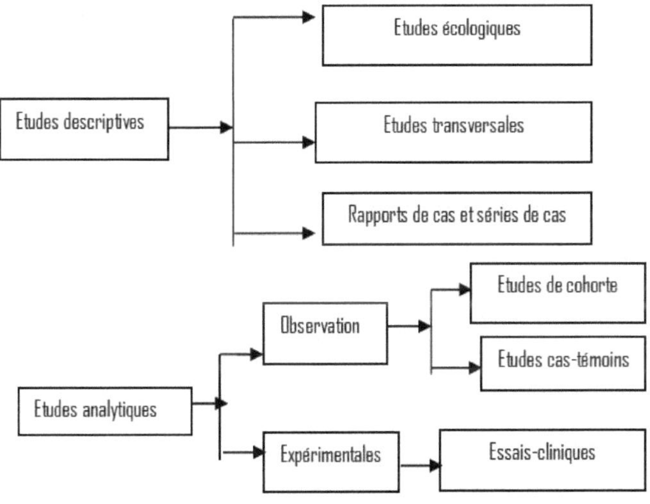

4.2 DESCRIPTIVE EPIDEMIOLOGY

4.2.1 Definition

Descriptive epidemiology describes the frequency and distribution of disease or health problems in populations as a function of person, place and time variables (Simpson et al., 2008).

4.2.2 Characteristics of a descriptive study

It describes and generates hypotheses and never tests hypotheses.

Descriptive studies consist in systematically collecting and analyzing data with a view to answering the following questions: What is the nature of the problem? How important is the problem? Who is affected? How do those affected by the problem behave? What do they think and know about the problem?

Descriptive studies deal with the distribution of problems: subgroups of the affected population, geographical distribution as well as variations in frequency over time. These studies can provide information that enables one or more epidemiological hypotheses to be formulated (OKITOLONDA 2015).

The descriptive study is not intended to test a hypothesis, but merely to provide information on the characteristics of a population (who? when? where?). This information may eventually lead to the formulation of a hypothesis, which must then be verified by an analytical study.

4.2.3 Questions answered by descriptive studies

Descriptive studies answer the questions: Who? Who? Where?

1°) <u>The individual</u> (who?)

Descriptive data about the individual corresponding to the question, "Who is sick?", age, gender, religion, marital status, personality type, race as well as socio-economic factors such as education, income and occupation.

2°) Location (where?)

The second question essentially posed by descriptive studies is "Where are the highest and lowest morbidity rates observed? Descriptive geographical features can provide important insights into the etiology of a disease.

3°) Time (when?)

The descriptive data concern the time corresponding to the questions "When is the disease most rare or most frequent?". In some respects, chronological changes in the rate of disease correspond to the classic concept of an epidemic, a significant increase in morbidity in a relatively short space of time.

4.2.4 Types of descriptive studies

There are three types of descriptive studies: case reports or case series, cross-sectional studies and ecological studies (Hennekens et all, 1998).

A. Case or case series observation reports

Follow an individual with a health problem, note the symptoms and formulate hypotheses, but never test them.

They involve the careful, detailed profiling of one or more patients by one or more doctors. Individual case studies can also be applied to case series, which give the characteristics of a number of patients suffering from a given disease. Case reports or case series are the most basic type of descriptive study: a patient or group of patients with the same diagnosis is followed, and hypotheses are formulated on the basis of a number of observations. Observations may represent the first signs of a new disease or risk factor, or the beginning of an outbreak. For example, it was a single case report that led to the hypothesis that the use of oral contraceptives increases the risk of venous thrombosis. Case studies represent an important interface between clinical medicine and epidemiology, and most often concern unusual clinical manifestations.

When carried out on a small scale, these studies are known as "descriptive case studies". A descriptive case study may focus on a single patient, a health facility or a village. A descriptive study may also be based on a series of cases.

Prevention is difficult, simply avoiding contact with the patient, as we don't know what the person is suffering from. The results are difficult to generalize. Prevalence cannot be calculated. There is no control group.

B. Cross-sectional studies (prevalence studies).

These are studies in which we look for the presence of a disease in an individual at a specific date (Hennekens et al., 1998). For example, health needs surveys. Cross-sectional studies are used to estimate the importance of a health problem and monitor its evolution, evaluate health interventions and formulate hypotheses. Cross-sectional studies, also known as prevalence studies, are commonly used in descriptive epidemiology to measure the prevalence of a disease.

Cross-sectional studies assess the current or past level of exposure. They describe an epidemiological picture and generate etiological hypotheses. The use of a survey questionnaire is one way of gathering information on exposure and disease. In prevalence studies, information on disease and exposure is obtained simultaneously, making it difficult to tell whether the disease preceded the exposure and vice versa. Short-term illnesses are also difficult to detect with prevalence. Thus, associations found between exposure or exposure levels and disease will better represent people with long-term illness. However, cross-sectional studies have the advantage of being relatively easy and less costly. Describe a health phenomenon and give its intensity, i.e. the number of cases in the population, and calculate its prevalence. This gives a snapshot of the situation, the intensity with which the problem is present in the population.

Advantages: fast, less expensive, generates assumptions ;

Disadvantage: difficult to tell whether the cause preceded the consequence (chronological sequence criterion).

C. Ecological studies (correlational study)

They are also known as correlational studies. Ecological studies differ from other observational epidemiological studies in that their method of analysis involves groups rather than individuals. These are studies in which the units of analysis are whole populations or groups rather than individuals, to describe the relationship between an exposure and a specific disease, or to describe a disease in relation to a factor of interest such as age, use of health services, etc. One group is therefore compared with another, and the results are compared with the results of other studies. One group is compared to another.

In general, geographic zones (countries, provinces, census areas, etc.) are used as units of analysis, and differences in exposures and outcomes of interest between these zones are compared. For example, we can study the association between median income and cancer mortality by province in Canada. This involves describing and hypothesizing from the correlations identified. Here, the study units are groups, unlike previous studies where the units were individuals.

Ex: average age at death in relation to average income of Lemba commune residents.

4.3 ANALYTICAL EPIDEMIOLOGY

4.3.1 Definition

Analytical epidemiology refers to studies designed to examine associations, usually presumed or hypothetical causal relationships. An analytical study generally aims to define or measure the effects of risk factors, or it may focus on the health effects of particular exposures.

4.3.2 Types of analytical studies

Analytical epidemiology includes observational and experimental analytical studies, i.e. clinical trials (preventive and therapeutic trials).

4.3.2.1 Observational analytical studies

In epidemiology, there are two types of analytical observational studies: cohort studies and case-control studies.

4.3.2.1.1 Cohort studies: longitudinal, follow-up and incidence studies (prospective studies)

Originally, the word cohort was used to designate a section of the population born during a given period. Over time, the meaning of the word has broadened to encompass any group of people followed or studied over a given period. Thus, we might speak of the cohort of women who had their first child in 2000, or the cohort of health studies students who took the epidemiology course in 2015.

A cohort study is designed to follow over time a closed dynamic population (closed cohort) of subjects who are initially unaffected by the event under study, with subjects who are already ill being ineligible.

Eligible subjects are assigned to different exposure groups at the start of the study (E^+ and E^-).

This "at-risk" population is followed for a defined period of time ("follow-up"), during or at the end of which the incident events sought are identified (new cases of disease or death). At the end of follow-up, subjects can be classified into four categories:

- Presentations of the incident ;
- Presentations that did not include the incident event ;
- Presentations of the incident ;
- Unexposed who did not present the incident event.

Cohort studies represent the most rigorous form of non-experimental epidemiological studies. They are the only way to assess the incidence of a disease, to establish a cause-and-effect relationship between risk factor and disease with the least possible bias, and to evaluate latency and relative risk with maximum precision.

However, the accuracy and validity of the information provided are obtained at the cost of an often considerable investment in time and resources, and cohort studies, like all other epidemiological studies, are subject to specific shortcomings that can taint their validity.

A cohort study is generally prospective and, in this case, useful for testing causal hypotheses.

However, a cohort study can also be retrospective, particularly when the expected event is rare or when its occurrence is preceded by a long latency period. In this case, it is easier to start the study when the exposure and outcome have already taken place, for example by exploiting available databases.

Advantages and weaknesses of cohort studies

- **Benefits**

- They establish the temporal consequence between exposure and the observed effect(s) (causality hypothesis);
- They are not subject to most of the biases affecting case-control studies:

  ✓ Retrospective risk factor measurement bias (recall bias),
  ✓ Selective survival bias;

- They are particularly suited to the study of common diseases;
- They can be used to calculate incidence, relative risk and other variables assessing the risk incurred by the exposed and unexposed population;
- They offer the advantage of being well suited to measuring the risk associated with certain exposure factors.

- **Weaknesses and drawbacks**

- They require the inclusion of a large number of subjects in the initial phase;
- They are not suitable for studying rare diseases, for which the number of subjects initially included would become prohibitive;
- They are time-consuming and very costly:
- They are not, therefore, exploratory studies: the hypotheses tested must first have acquired their scientific basis through lighter studies;

- They remain subject to the potential existence of selection bias, misclassification, or bias related to confounding factors;
- They are exposed to the possible presence of related to the loss of follow-up of the subjects included ;

Recommendations for selecting subjects for cohort surveys

What the control group provides us with in a cohort study is the expected frequency of the disease in a group comparable in all respects to the group exposed to the risk factor, except for the fact that they are not exposed to the factor under study.

In a cohort study, we want to be sure that unexposed subjects come from the same population as exposed subjects. Unexposed subjects must have the same theoretical risk of contracting the disease as exposed subjects if they were to come into contact with the risk factor.

Potential sources of exposed and unexposed subjects include

- General population
- General population sample
- Special groups (doctors, veterans, etc.)
- Professional groups with different levels of exposure.

Examples:

- In the general population, birth certificates are matched with death certificates for a given state. We can then determine the characteristics associated with the increased risk of death among infants;
- General population sample: we take a sample of people living in a certain city; we determine their tobacco consumption, their degree of obesity, their cholesterol

level, etc.... we follow them for several years to see if they develop cardiovascular disease (Framingham survey);

- Special groups: we take all Vietnam veterans and retrospectively determine their exposure to Agent Orange. We then look at the occurrence of premature lung cancer in the "exposed" and "non-exposed" groups;
- Occupational groups: we take miners from a uranium mine and determine their level of exposure to this product. They are monitored to see if they develop lung cancer (exposure to the risk factor is of variable intensity).

  Or we take uranium miners and follow them to see if they develop lung cancer; we compare lung cancer rates with those of the general population (non-exposed group).

4.3.2.1.2 Case-control studies

(We take the disease into account, i.e. we look for the origin of the disease because exposure has already occurred).

It is an analytical observational study in which subjects are selected according to the presence (cases) or absence (controls) of the disease under study. A case-control study is always retrospective, since it looks to the past for the possible cause of an effect. In a case-control study, the researcher selects two groups of subjects from the same "source population", and strives to increase comparability by controlling for major characteristics.

Case-control studies :

- Requires limited time and manpower,
- Are particularly suited to the study of rare events,
- This makes it easy to formulate new etiological hypotheses,

- Do not put subjects at risk.

They pose two major problems:

- Exposure is defined after the event has occurred,
- Cases and controls come from two populations that are never perfectly comparable, and biases are possible (selection bias, indication bias).

Case-control studies are indicated in the following circumstances:

1. rare disease in a population (prevalence rate < 5%)

2. when you don't want to put your subjects at risk

3. the disease is already present and we want to look for risk factors

Case-control studies can have the following advantages and disadvantages:

- **Advantages**: case-control studies offer the following advantages:

- It can be completed quickly. These studies are often of short duration. The disease has already been declared and the etiological investigation is usually retrospective. The duration of the study is independent of the incubation or latency period.

- The case-control strategy is particularly interesting for rare diseases,

- A case-control study enables us to gather a sufficient number of sick subjects to make statistically satisfactory comparisons of the distribution of risk factors between patients and healthy subjects. Fewer subjects are required, as the study is based on previously reported cases.

- In a case-control study, we can analyze a large number of presumed risk factors collected from the subjects' histories.

- A case-control study is therefore much less costly in terms of agents, time and personnel.

- A case-control study makes it possible to investigate even the harmful effects of a drug or product, whereas there would be ethical problems if the study were carried out prospectively. Here, the study subjects are not put at risk.

➢ **The disadvantages** of case-control studies are as follows:

- Inherent risk of bias in control selection (often in hospital settings)

- Desired information may not be available in medical records or when memory is called upon;

- Difficulties (impossibility) of determining incidence and attack rates in exposed and unexposed populations;

- Information provided by the case where the control is likely to be biased. Case-control studies are particularly prone to selection and recall bias. Indeed, the case may remember factors in the past better than the control, especially for serious diseases such as AIDS, leukemia, cancer, etc.

- Difficulties in accurately and precisely defining exposure;

A. Case selection

One of the first elements to be considered in a case-control study is the definition of the disease or event being studied. The definition of the disease must be a homogeneous entity, hence the need to determine specific and precise disease criteria (definite cases, probable cases, possible cases). Cases can be identified using a screening questionnaire with a specific question on a history of asthma, for example, diagnosed by a doctor (possible asthma diagnosis). Objective tests such as the allergy skin test or the methacholine bronchial provocation test can also be used (probable diagnosis). Finally, cases can be defined on the basis of clinical examination (definitive diagnosis of asthma).

Precise inclusion and exclusion criteria must also be established for cases. For example, you may decide to work on cases aged 20-45 years for asthma (to exclude chronic obstructive pulmonary disease (emphysema - chronic bronchitis), belonging to a given ethnic group (if you suspect that the disease is associated with a particular ethnic group), and so on.

Case recruitment sources can be hospitals (hospital-based), private clinics, case registries (cancer, or notifiable disease) or the general population. Hospital-based cases are easy to recruit and relatively less costly. However, it is difficult to generalize results from these cases to the general population if the recruiting hospital is a tertiary or specialist hospital. Cases selected from the general population are expensive, but their results are easily generalizable if all cases have been identified. If only a small proportion of cases in the general population have been identified, it will be very difficult to say how representative these are of all possible cases.

B. Witness selection

This is undoubtedly the most difficult and most criticized stage in the design of a case-control study.

In selecting controls, we must consider certain characteristics of the cases, their origin, the possibility of obtaining information of the same quality as in the cases, and the cost of this operation. Controls must also meet the same inclusion and/or exclusion criteria as cases.

Like the cases, the witnesses may be hospital-based or geographical. Witnesses can also be relatives, spouses or friends of cases. Hospital-based controls have the advantage of being easy to recruit, i.e. at low cost and with little effort. With hospital controls, there are low refusal rates, and the controls are as aware as the cases of their previous exposures. This reduces the risk of memory bias. Hospitalized controls also have advantages because, being ill, they differ from the general population and have characteristics associated with being hospitalized. The causes of hospitalization of hospitalized controls should be varied and with no known relationship to the exposure and disease under study. The consequences of these disadvantages are the underestimation of cigarette smoking on the incidence of bladder cancer, as the frequency of smoking is high among hospitalized controls.

Geographic or population-based controls come from the same catchment area. They are generally of better quality than hospital-based controls. They are recruited by "door-to-door" canvassing in the selected area, by telephone calls (with numbers chosen at random), or by using census or electoral lists. Difficulties in recruiting geographic controls are mainly related to obtaining lists and contacting subjects. In addition, people in good health show little interest in taking part in the study. Finally, the quality of information provided by healthy controls is sometimes of questionable quality. We must always ask ourselves whether the subjects who agree to take part are different from the general population in terms of the risk factors studied.

Spouses, family members, immediate neighbors or people living in the same electoral district as the cases can be witnesses. They have the advantages of willing participation, less memory bias and greater ease in meeting the study's requirements concerning factors such as environment, socioeconomic status, ethnic group, etc. However, these controls have the enormous disadvantage of being more likely to share certain exposures (such as diet, consumption of contaminated water, etc.) with the cases.

Controls can be selected randomly or systematically (from a list where, for example, all the eighth subjects are chosen) and according to time constraints (for example, the control is chosen within one month of case recruitment).

Table 8: Comparison of cohort, case-control and cross-sectional studies (Olivier Degomme 2010)

Types of study	Benefits	Disadvantages
Cross-sectional study	Low cost Fast	No notion of time No idea of causality
Case-control study	Low cost Fast Moderate sample size	No impact Memory/selection bias No RR
Cohort study	Little memory/selection bias	High cost Long latency period Ethical issues

C) Potential sources of cases and witnesses

Control cases

- Community Community
- Clinical Clinical
- Hospital Hospital
- Neighborhood register

Friends

Family members Other reference groups available outside the survey

<u>Examples</u>:

- Investigating the monkeypox epidemic
  Case: Community; Witnesses: family members

Hospital-acquired streptococcal infection

Cases: hospital; controls: same hospital

- Toxic shock syndrome

Cases: hospital; controls: friends

- Ovarian cancer

Case: Register; Witness: Community

- Angiosarcoma of the liver

Case: register; witness: neighborhood

4.3.2.2 Analytical intervention studies

4.3.2.2.1 Experimental studies

A. Characteristics of an experimental study

Experimental studies are clinical trials.

An experimental study has three characteristics

- 2 groups ;
- The researcher organizes exposure to the factor under study (factor manipulation);
- The researcher organizes the random allocation of exposure, of the factor studied, to the subjects, who are thus divided into two groups: the experimental group and the control group. This procedure is called "**randomization**".

Example

- Laboratory test to evaluate the response of individuals to a situation, a stimulation, imposed by the research protocol;
- Comparison of one treatment and placebo, comparison of two treatments ;
- Exposure of subjects to a preventive intervention, which seeks to reduce risk (Fluoride and prevention of dental caries, iodine and prevention of iodine deficiency disorders, evaluation of the efficacy of a new vaccine, evaluation of the efficacy of a diagnostic procedure, etc.).

Clinical trials are the most common form of trial. Typically, a randomized controlled trial (RCT) is designed to test new or existing methods of treatment or intervention for particular diseases in people who have those diseases. By design, clinical trials assess the efficacy of one treatment versus another (by controlling for factors that might affect the association between the treatment and the expected effect). Clinical trials are divided into therapeutic and prevention trials.

Therapeutic trials are carried out on groups of patients suffering from a particular disease, with the aim of determining the effectiveness of a treatment in making symptoms more visible, preventing relapse and reducing the death rate. Prevention trials are carried out in populations of healthy subjects at normal or high risk of developing a disease. In both cases, the principle is to hold constant, as far as possible, all factors except the treatment or intervention.

Clinical trials can pose problems of ethics (if knowledge of the new treatment is not too advanced and if there is insufficient data on the potential beneficial effects of the treatment), feasibility and cost. Ethical problems may also arise if knowledge of the beneficial effects is sufficiently advanced. In such cases, it would be unethical to deprive patients in the control group of this intervention.

During trials, non-adherence may occur because of side effects (e.g. increased weight, nausea, dizziness, etc.), increased disease severity or failure to take the treatment.

CHAPTER 5: DISEASE FREQUENCY MEASUREMENT

In epidemiology, the two fundamental measures of frequency are prevalence and incidence. These concepts can be approached by considering the natural history of the disease.

Consider a given population. At any given moment, each individual is characterized by a particular state of health, which theoretically allows him or her to be located in one of the "boxes" used to represent this state (e.g., "uninfected", "infected not sick", "sick contagious", etc.).

5.1 PREVALENCE

Prevalence is a measure of the frequency of this condition at a given time. It is a measure of the presence of the disease, or more generally of the presence of some characteristic, in the population. It is the number of people affected by a health problem over a given period. This is called a cross-sectional measure, as it provides information on the situation at the time of measurement. Here, we're already sick.

In this population, during any given time interval, a variable number of individuals move from one state to another (for example, a susceptible individual becomes infected, an infected individual becomes ill, etc.).

Prevalence is a proportion, although the term "prevalence rate" is often misused.

The term "prevalence" refers to a proportion that varies from 0 to 1 and has no units. However, prevalence is usually expressed by multiplying the observed proportion by a unit of size (100, 1000, 100,000, etc., depending on the case). This avoids the need to handle decimals and makes the value of the calculated ratio more concrete.

Marmite of Prevalence

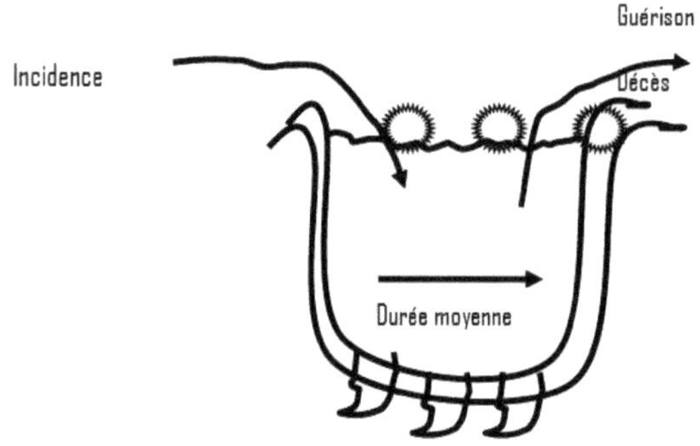

The numerator of this proportion includes all subjects with the characteristic under study at the time of measurement. Defining the numerator requires the use of precise, uniform criteria to define cases, and rigorous control to avoid observation errors. The denominator comprises all the subjects in the study population, i.e. the sick and the non-diseased. As with the numerator, defining the denominator requires a precise count of the population under study.

There is a relationship between prevalence and incidence: Prevalence = Incidence × Duration

- *Many new cases (Incidence ↑) →short duration of disease: prevalence ↓*
- *Chronic illness: →duration of long illness: prevalence ↑*

5.1.1 Prevalence function

Prevalence has two main functions: epidemiological and operational. In its epidemiological function, prevalence is used to measure the dimension of health problems at a given time (the number of people affected by the health problem), and to compare disease frequencies in different groups, as a function of place or time. In its operational aspect, prevalence is mainly used in health planning, as it is a good estimator of health needs and services.

5.1.2 Types of prevalence

Two types of prevalence are distinguished: instantaneous prevalence (IP) and period prevalence (PP).

5.1.2.1 Instantaneous prevalence (IP).

Instantaneous prevalence is the number of people affected by a disease or attribute at a given moment in time, divided by the total population at that moment.

$$PI = \frac{\text{Tous les cas actuels d'une maladie à un moment donné}}{\text{Total de la population étudiée à ce moment}}$$

Example: on 18/05/2018, 20,0000 students on the university site, the survey identifies 250 students with malaria at 12:30 pm.

$$\text{P.I} = \frac{250}{20.000} = 13\ pour\ milles$$

This prevalence may change in the following hours.

5.1.2.2 Period prevalence (PP).

Period prevalence is a hybrid concept, combining the notions of prevalence and incidence. The numerator is equal to the sum of prevalent cases at time 0 and new incident cases over the period from time 0 to time 1. It is equal to the number of people who have been affected by a disease or presented with an attribute at any time during a specific observation period, divided by the size of the population at the start of said observation period.

$$PP = \frac{\text{Tout les cas d'unemaladie au cours d'unepériode précise}}{\text{Total de la population au début de ladite période}}$$

The numerator is equal to the sum of prevalent cases at time 0 and new incident cases over the period from time 0 to time 1. The denominator is equal to the population at time 0, if the population is stable, or to the number of subjects observed during the period, if the population is unstable.

Example: January 1st 10,000 people and December 31st 12,000 people, a 12-month period. During this period there were 150 cases of illness.

$$P.P = \frac{150}{10.000} = 15 \textit{pour milles}$$

5.2 THE IMPACT

Incidence is a measure of the frequency of the "becoming ill" event over a given period of time. Incidence measures the number of new cases of a particular disease or event in the population at risk over a known period of time. It is a measure of new cases of disease.

5.2.1 Types of impact

There are two types of incidence measurement: cumulative incidence and incidence rate.

5.2.1.1 Cumulative incidence (CI) or incidence proportion (for a closed cohort).

Cumulative incidence measures the number of people who become ill (or suffer a health event) during the observation period in a population at risk. The calculation of cumulative incidence assumes two conditions: all subjects at risk are free of the disease studied at the start of the follow-up period (otherwise, the measurement reverts to the calculation of period prevalence) and all subjects at risk at the start of the follow-up period are effectively followed through to the end, i.e. the withdrawals observed during the follow-up period were caused by the disease or event studied. If this condition is not met, there is a risk of underestimating the cumulative incidence, since incident cases will escape registration. This is the probability of becoming ill when exposed. It is a conditional probability (A→B : exposed → ill).

Cumulative incidence is calculated by dividing "the number of new cases of a disease over a given period of time by the total population at risk".

$$IC = \frac{\text{Nombre nouveaux cas d'une maladie au cours d'unepériode de temps donnée}}{\text{population totale soumise au risque}}$$

Population at risk: this is the population at the start of the period, i.e. when the cohort was being set up.

Cumulative incidence is expressed without any particular unit, in per 100, per 1,000, and so on. However, cumulative incidence is impossible to interpret without precise information on the length of the observation period. A cumulative incidence of death equal to 3% may be considered small if the observation period is 20 years, whereas it will be considered significant if the observation period is 20 years.

Cumulative incidence is an estimate of the probability or risk, for an individual, of developing a disease over a given period of time. Cumulative incidence measures the conditional probability of an event occurring. A conditional probability measures the likelihood of one event occurring when another has already taken place.

Cumulative incidence is an indicator with an epidemiological function. As it is a direct measure of individual risk over an observation period of known duration, it is useful for determining prognosis. It lends itself particularly well to "survival" analysis, i.e. the calculation of probabilities of "occurrence" or "non-occurrence" of any dichotomous event: death and survival, disease and non-disease, cure and non-healing, etc.

Cumulative incidence also has an operational function. It enables us to compare the effectiveness of procedures or programs implemented to control the event under study. If this effectiveness is real, the risk of incidental events decreases.

5.2.2.2 Incidence rate (IR): (for an open cohort).

The incidence rate measures the rate of spread of a disease in a population at risk. It is indicated for the open population, in which entries (births and immigration) and exits (deaths and emigration) are observed. The incidence rate is equal to the number of people who become new cases of the disease divided by the number of time-persons at risk.

$$\text{TI} = \frac{\text{Nombre de nouveaux cas}}{\text{personnes} - \text{temps à risque}}$$

Person-time at risk: this is the time spent by each individual in the cohort. We speak of person-week, person-month, person-year.

Example 1: An individual at risk of disease, under observation since July 1er and remaining at risk until December 31 of the same year, has accumulated six months or 184 days at risk. This person counts as 184 person-days at risk.

Figure 4.1 Example of incidence rate (IR) calculation

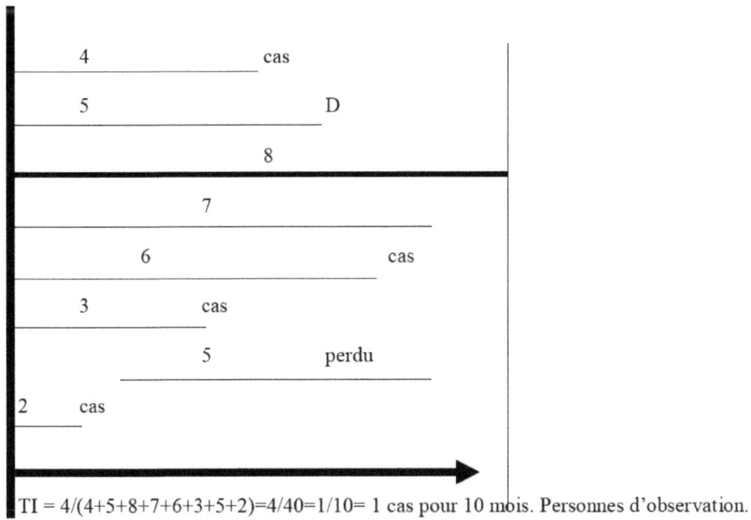

The numerator is the same as that used to calculate cumulative incidence. It's the number of people who go from not being a case to being a case, or, more precisely, from not having experienced the expected event to having experienced it. The denominator of the incidence rate is expressed in complex units: person-time (PT) at risk. This concept measures both the number of people exposed and, for each of them, the length of time they are exposed during the observation period.

Example:

An individual at risk of disease, under observation since January 1er and remaining at risk until December 31 of the same year, has accumulated twelve months or 365 days of risk. He is counted in the denominator, for 365 person-days. Another individual, also under observation since July 1er , fell ill on October 1er and, of course, once ill, is no longer at risk (unless it's a benign event of negligible duration, such as a cold or superficial injury). This subject's period of exposure to risk therefore ends when the illness appears, and lasts exactly three months or 92 days. This patient is included in the denominator for 92 person-days.

The exact calculation of person-time is made by adding together the exact durations of exposure to risk for each of the people observed.

$$PT = \sum (ni + dti)$$

As the contribution of each subject to the observation is often difficult to specify, an approximate person-time calculation can be made by multiplying the half-time of the populations at the beginning and end of the observation period.

$$PT = [(No + Nt) /2] * dt$$

The exact calculation of person-time is made by adding together the exact durations of exposure to risk for each of the people observed.

A sample exercise:

Over a ten-year period, 350 cases of work-related injuries were recorded among factory employees. The number of plant employees was 320 at the start of the injury recording period and 480 at the end.

What frequency measurement can be calculated here? Perform the calculation.

Solution:

Since the population is open (320 people at the start of the study and 480 at the end), we need to **calculate the incidence rate.**

a) First, we calculate an average population: (480 + 320) /2 = 800/2 = 400 people
b) We calculate the total number of person-years: 400 persons * 10 = 4000 person-years;
c) The incidence rate is calculated: 350 (No. of new cases) /4000 = 0.09 cases/person-year. (Work-related injuries occur at a rate of 0.09 cases per person-year over the 10 years of the study).

The incidence rate has an **epidemiological function.** It is not a direct estimator of individual risk, since each individual follow-up time is only a fraction of the total risk exposure time for a given individual. Rather, the incidence rate provides information on short-term risk for a time interval that tends towards zero, i.e., information on the transmission and dynamics of the disease. This information can be used to characterize a group of people, and is particularly useful in etiological research.

The incidence rate has the same **operational function** as the cumulative incidence. It makes it possible to compare the effectiveness of certain procedures or programs implemented to control the event under study.

5.3 MORTALITY MEASUREMENTS

Since death is an irreversible individual event, all mortality measures are variants of incidence measures. Their importance, however, warrants more detailed consideration.

The main mortality measures are of the same two types as incidence measures: lethality measures and death rate measures.

To these two mortality measures we must add a set of indices used to monitor maternity and early childhood problems.

5.3.1 Lethality

Lethality is a particular form of cumulative incidence, measuring the number of people who die from a disease within the population of people who become ill. Lethality can be calculated for all causes combined, or specifically (cause-specific lethality). Lethality measures the conditional probability of dying when one becomes ill:

Lethality = Pro (deaths/M+) or

$$= \frac{\text{Nombre de décès attribuables à une maladie donnée durant une période}}{\text{Nombre de personnes souffrant de cette maladie durant la même période}}$$

Lethality is a proportion, but common usage authorizes the use of the term "lethality rate".

Lethality is an indicator used to determine individual risk of death and to perform survival analyses. This indicator can be used to formulate a prognosis, which is particularly useful when comparing two different treatments designed to prolong survival.

5.3.2 Mortality rate

The crude death rate takes into account all deaths occurring in the population without distinguishing between groups of subjects. As such, it is not a very useful measure, as it is strongly influenced by the age structure of the population.

$$\text{Overall mortality } x = \frac{\text{Nombre de décès total pendant une période}}{\text{Population étudiée pendant la période}}$$

The **specific mortality rate** takes into account differences between groups of subjects. A specific rate can be calculated by disease, by age, by sex, for another characteristic deemed important, or any combination of these factors. It is these specific rates that enable comparisons to be made.

Specific mortality

For a given cause = $\frac{\text{Nombre de décès dus à cette cause pendant une période}}{\text{Population étudiée pendant la période}}$

Specific mortality for a given age group

= $\frac{\text{Nombre de décès dans cette classe d'âgependant une période}}{\text{Population totala étudiée pendant la période}}$

The **proportional mortality rate** represents the proportion of deaths due to a given cause out of all deaths observed during a given period.

Proportional mortality

Cause-related = $\frac{\text{Nombre de décès dus à cette cause pendant une période}}{\text{Totalité de décès pendant la période}}$

Age and mortality

Age has a major influence on mortality. Before comparing the mortality of 2 groups, we must first take into account the composition of the population in the two groups. This is important because the group where young people predominate may have a lower overall mortality rate than the group where older people predominate 3ème . Age can thus constitute a 3ème factor commonly referred to in epidemiology as a confounding factor. This is why it is essential to adjust rates according to the composition of the population.

Age-specific mortality and standardization

It is often advisable to calculate the mortality rate for each age group to allow for adjustment. The age-specific mortality rate adjustment is calculated as follows:

Age-specific mortality x proportion of population by age group

Example: suppose we want to compare the mortality rates of 2 communities, community A and community B.

The population of community A is 50% young and 50% old. Specific mortality rates are 4/1000 and 16/1000 respectively. The population of community B is 67% young and 33% old, with specific mortality rates of 5/1000 and 20/1000 respectively. Thus the general mortality rate in community A will be (4 x 0.5) + (16 x0.5) = 10/1000 and in community B (5 x 0.67) + (20 x 0.33) = 10/1000.

Looking at these rates, we get the impression that the 2 communities have similar general mortality rates. This impression is erroneous, as we'll see once we've taken the age factor into account.

Adjusting the mortality rates for the 2 communities gives us the following two rates:

N.B: we'll adjust the mortality rate using community B as a reference, so we'll multiply the specific mortality rates of the 2 communities a and B by the fractions of the population composition of community B.

A: (4) (0.67) + (16) (0.33) = 8.9 per 1000

B: (5) (0.67) + (20) (0.33) = 10 per 1000

Thus, the 2 communities after adjustment have different mortality rates. We have thus removed the effect of age composition, enabling us to make valid comparisons.

Table 9: **Exercise**: the following malaria data are available for two regions over a one-year period.

	Region 1	Region 2
Population	125 254	15987
New cases of malaria	4569	1749
Total number of deaths	2453	556
Number of deaths due to malaria.	650	520
For men		
Total malaria cases	4800	4750
Number of deaths due to malaria.	569	217

Calculate for each year and for each region :

1) Malaria incidence per 1,000 inhabitants = $\frac{4569}{125\ 254}$ x 1000 = 36

2) Malaria prevalence per 1,000 inhabitants = $\frac{4800}{125\ 254}$ x 1000 = 38

3) Crude mortality per 1,000 inhabitants = $\frac{2453}{125254} \times 1000 =$ 19,5

4) Specific mortality per 1,000 inhabitants = $\frac{650}{125\ 254} \times 1000 = 5$

   For men

5) Proportional mortality rate due to malaria per 1,000 inhabitants

   $= \frac{569}{2453} \times 1000 = 232$

6) Malaria case-fatality rate per 1,000 inhabitants

$$= \frac{569}{4800} \times 1000 \; = 118 \sim 119$$

CHAPTER 6: ASSOCIATION MEASURES IN EPIDEMIOLOGY

INTRODUCTION

Measures of association are useful when assessing the strength of the relationship between two or more variables (exposure and the health problems under study). The most frequently used measures of association specific to epidemiology are relative risk (RR), attributable risk (AR) and odds ratio (OR), which in certain circumstances is an approximation of relative risk. AR is also known as an impact measure, because it aims to quantify the effect of a particular factor on the frequency of disease. If the effect is negative, we measure the etiological fraction of the risk; if the effect is positive, we measure the preventable fraction.

Relative risk (RR) and attributable risk (AR) are the two measures of association between an exposure factor (E) and an outcome that are frequently calculated in epidemiology.

Relative risk (RR) or (risk ratio): this is the ratio between the incidence (risk) in the exposed population and the incidence (risk) in the unexposed population.

Attributable risk (risk difference): this is the difference between the risk (incidence) in the exposed population and the risk (incidence) in the unexposed population. It is the proportion of risk actually attributable to the exposure concerned.

To facilitate the calculation of measures of association, researchers often present epidemiological data in a two-by-two table, also known as a contingency table. This table contains four cells (a, b, c and d). Each of these cells represents the number of individuals corresponding to a combination of exposure and disease state.

- a = E+ D+, exposed subjects who have become ill ;
- b = E+ D-, exposed subjects remain unharmed ;
- c = E- D+, unexposed subjects who became ill ;
- d = E- D-, unexposed subjects remain unharmed.

The various totals for these cells are (in number of subjects, if cumulative incidence is involved, and in person-time at risk, if incidence totals are involved):

- (a+b) = total number of exposures ;
- (c+d) = total non-exposed ;
- (a+c) = total number of incident cases or people with the disease ;
- (b+d) = the total number of subjects free of the disease under study ;
- (a+b+c+d) = the total number of subjects or time-persons in the study.

Table 10: Presentation of a two-by-two array

Exhibition	**Disease**		
	Yes	No	Total
Yes	A	B	a+b
No	C	D	c+d
Total	a+c	b+d	a+b+c+d

To illustrate the construction of a two-by-two table, the following table uses (fictitious) data from a cohort study on the association between depression and the later development of dementia in young adults. Following the follow-up of 15,200 patients aged 18 to 20, this study revealed 630 cases of depression, 23 of which subsequently developed dementia. The study also revealed 79 cases of dementia in the 14,570 patients who had never experienced depression. On the basis of these data, it would be possible to construct the table as follows:

Table 11: Presentation of data from a cohort study on the association between Depression and the later development of dementia in young adults

Depression	Dementia		**Total**
	Yes	No	
Yes	23	607	630
No	79	14491	14570
Total	102	15098	15200

6.1 RELATIVE RISK

Relative risk (RR) is the ratio of disease incidence in exposed subjects to that in unexposed subjects. It answers the question: how many times more likely are exposed subjects to contract the disease than unexposed subjects?

- *Incidence (Risk) among the exposed = Re+ = a/(a+b)*
- *Incidence (Risk) among the unexposed = Re- = c/(c+d)*

$$RR = (a/a+b)/(c/c+d)$$

For example, in the study of the association between depression and the later development of dementia in young adults, the RR is calculated as follows:

$$RR = (23/630) / (79/14570)$$

$$= 0{,}036/0{,}005$$

$$= 7{,}20$$

If RR = 1: the numerator equals the denominator, and the incidence of disease in the exposed group equals the incidence of disease in the unexposed group. In this case, the risks are the same in both groups.

If RR>1: this indicates a positive association between the risk factor and the disease (the numerator is greater than the denominator), meaning that there is a higher risk in subjects exposed than in those not exposed to the risk factor concerned.

Thus, the RR calculated above indicates a risk 7 times higher in young adults who have experienced depression than in those who have never experienced depression.

If RR < 1: there is a negative association between the risk factor and the disease (the numerator is lower than the denominator), i.e. a lower risk in exposed subjects than in unexposed subjects. In this case, exposure may have a protective effect against the disease.

6.2 ATTRIBUTABLE RISK (AR):

(Risk difference): this is the difference between the risk (incidence) in the exposed and the risk (incidence) in the unexposed. It is the proportion of the risk actually attributable to the exposure concerned.

The AR gives the dimension of the public health problem posed by a risk factor, and provides an estimate of the public health gain to be expected if the risk factor is eliminated. AR can therefore be a useful measure of the impact of a given exposure on public health.

$$RA = (a/a+b) - (c/c+d)$$

Returning to our example of the study of the association between depression and the later development of dementia in young adults, we calculate the AR as follows:

$$RA = (23/630) - (79/14570)$$

$$= 0{,}036 - 0{,}005)$$

$$= 0{,}031$$

The number of cases of dementia attributable to depression is 31 per 1,000 inhabitants.

The RA therefore assumes that there is a causal relationship between exposure and disease. The RA is 0 if there is no association between exposure and the health problem. If there is a causal association between exposure and health problem, the AR is greater than 0.

To estimate the proportion of disease cases attributable to exposure in exposed subjects, or the proportion that could be avoided by eliminating exposure, AR is often expressed as a percentage (AR%). The percentage of attributable risk, or attributable percentage, or ecological fraction is calculated by multiplying by 100 the result of the ratio between the attributable risk and the incidence of disease in exposed subjects.

$$RA\ \% = (RA/Ie) * 100$$

With our example on the study of the association between depression and dementia, we will have :

$$RA\% = 0.031/(23/630) * 100$$

$$= 0{,}8491 * 100$$

$$= 84{,}91\%$$

In fact, nearly 85% of dementia cases in this cohort are attributable to depression. Preventing depression in this cohort could therefore prevent 85% of dementia cases.

Table 12: Types of study, measures of frequency and measures of association

Types of study	Frequency measurement	Association measures
Cross-sectional study (cross-sectional study)	Prevalence of exposure Prevalence in unexposed individuals	Prevalence ratio (PR) = Relative Risk (RR)
Case-control study (case-control study)	% exposure in cases % exposure in controls	Odds Radio (OR) =Relative Risk (RR) (low prevalence)
Cohort study (cohort sudy)	Incidence of exposure Incidence in unexposed individuals	Relative Risk (RR)

CHAPTER 7. EPIDEMIC INVESTIGATION AND SURVEILLANCE

7.1 INVESTIGATING EPIDEMICS

These are epidemiological methods for controlling, eradicating and monitoring epidemics.

The evolution in time and space of a disease in a given community is a function of a delicate balance between a multitude of factors that facilitate or prevent its spread. These factors include variations in the composition of the population according to the different characteristics of individuals, variations in environmental conditions and changes in the properties of the pathogen.

Epidemiological control of each contagious process is achieved in several ways, the main ones being: control, eradication and epidemiological surveillance.

7.1.1 Conditions for an epidemic to develop

Epidemics do not happen by chance: they are linked to an ecological context, characterized by an imbalance, at a given moment, between the disease agent and the host, in the presence of a suitable mode of transmission;

The factors necessary for the development and persistence of an epidemic are :

- The presence of a pathogen in sufficient quantity (reservoir);
- Not enough people are both receptive and exposed to this agent;
- The existence of an appropriate mode of transmission between this agent and receptive individuals, making contamination possible. The environment must be conducive to this mode of transmission.

7.1.2 Mode of transmission of the causal agent

1. Main modes of transmission of the causal agent

There are two main modes of transmission of the causative agent:

a) **Cross-transmission, from person to person :**

- Either directly, as in the case of inter-human transmission of tuberculosis by air: This occurs through the inhalation of droplets of bronchial secretions emitted by the tuberculosis patient when he coughs;

- Either via an intermediary (vector) such as hands, or contaminated equipment (e.g. transmission of HIV between drug users via contaminated needles), or an insect (malaria is transmitted from patient to patient via mosquitoes that suck up and then reinject blood contaminated with the malaria parasite).

b) Transmission from a common reservoir

For example: consumption of contaminated food or water responsible for gastroenteritis.

Controlling an epidemic requires an understanding of the factors related to the micro-organism, the host and the environment that enabled a sufficient level of transmission to cause the epidemic.

2. importance of knowing the mode of transmission of the causal agent

Knowledge of the causal agent's mode of transmission is essential, as interrupting the epidemic requires breaking this chain at at least one point:

. *Eliminate the pathogen reservoir :*

- Destruction of foodstuffs contaminated by bacteria;
- Disinfection of drinking water ;
- Sanitation and environmental hygiene for water- and food-borne diseases;
- Eviction from school for contagious childhood diseases;
- Treatment of infected patients likely to constitute a reservoir for new cases, etc.

. *Or reduce the host's susceptibility :*

- Prophylactic treatment,
- Vaccination,
- Gamma globulin immunotherapy for measles, rubella, meningococcal meningitis, etc.

. Or block the transmission process, for example :

- Observance of basic hygiene measures (hand washing),
- Respect for the cold chain,
- Case isolation,
- Mosquito control, etc.

These possibilities are not mutually exclusive.

7.1.3 Investigating an epidemic

To investigate an epidemic, follow these steps:

1°) Establish the existence of the epidemic and define the disease, take the first practical steps

- Case definition
- Several similar cases
- Laboratory confirmation
- Apply initial measures to control transmission and manage cases

2°) Confirming the epidemic

- Identify all cases
- Increase in the number of cases compared with the usual situation
- High number of observed cases compared to expected number of cases

3°) Characterizing cases

- Represent the distribution of cases spatially (mapping) and temporally
- This means finding answers to the following questions: Where? When? Who?
- Identify at-risk populations, i.e. answer the question of what are the characteristics of these people.

4°) Building the epidemic curve

The epidemic curve describes the occurrence of cases in an epidemic episode as a function of time. It is represented by a histogram or curve plotted by plotting time periods or intervals on the x-axis, and the number of cases occurring during each time period on the y-axis. The choice of time unit depends on the incubation period of the disease. In order to obtain an epidemic curve that is neither too spread out nor too compressed, we choose a time unit roughly equal to a quarter of the incubation period of the disease, where this is known.

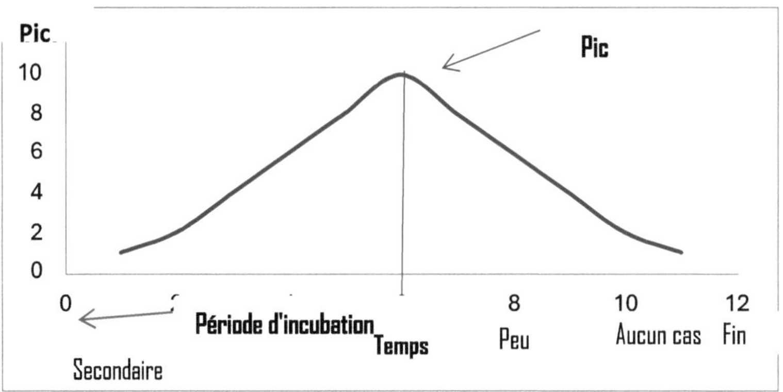

If the disease in question is not known, the average incubation period for this disease can be determined using the epidemic curve. This is the period from the first case (index case) to the peak of the epidemic curve.

a) Description of the epidemic curve

We systematically examine

- Epidemic start date or time: d_{mi}
- Epidemic end date or time: d_{fin}
- The number of cases
- Total duration of the epidemic :
- The presence of one or more peaks
- Peak date(s): d_{pic}
- The existence of outliers
- The general profile of the curve

b) Interpreting the epidemic curve

Interpretation of the curve could enable us to develop hypotheses on the nature of the causal agent of the epidemic episode, its source and mode of transmission.

The shape of an epidemic curve can provide information on the nature of the source.

Common point source: the epidemic curve is unimodal (a single peak), with a rapid rise and a slight fall off to the right. In this case, there is a close clustering of cases, as many individuals are contaminated by the same source at the same time. For example, contamination by the same food or drink consumed by a group of people during a brief exposure. Using such a curve, it is possible to pinpoint the period of exposure to the source.

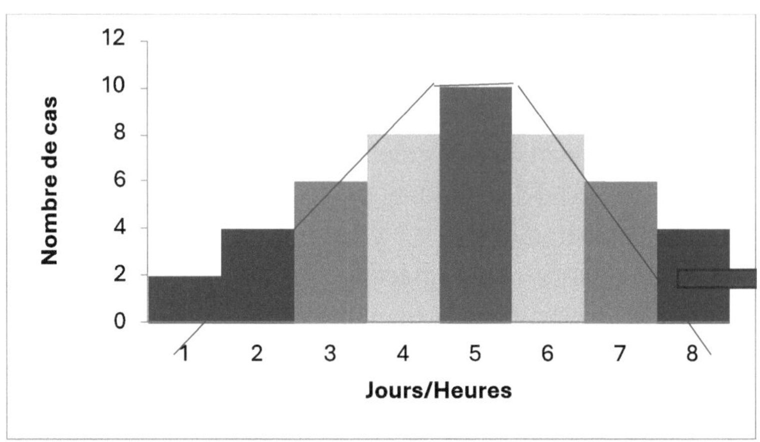

Example: Contamination from a meal or drink

Persistent source: a curve with a rapid rise, followed by a plateau, is observed when the source of the epidemic is persistent in the community.

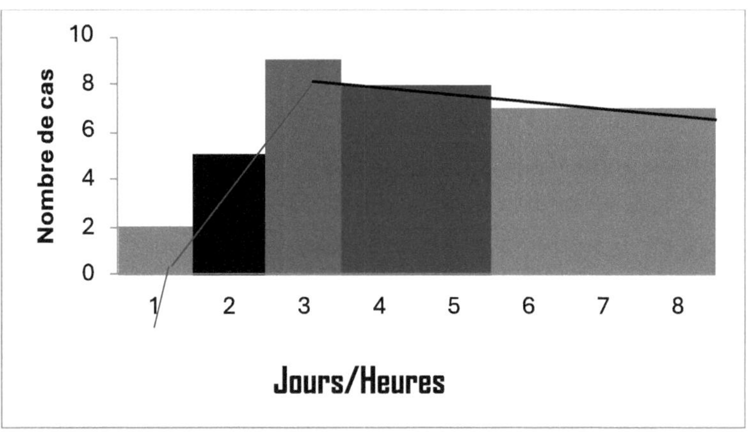

Example: Cholera epidemic in Goma

Human-to-human or person-to-person transmission: this takes the form of a curve showing an initial gentle rise, followed by several waves of increasing amplitude, reflecting the contamination of groups of individuals by close contact, and a slow decline.

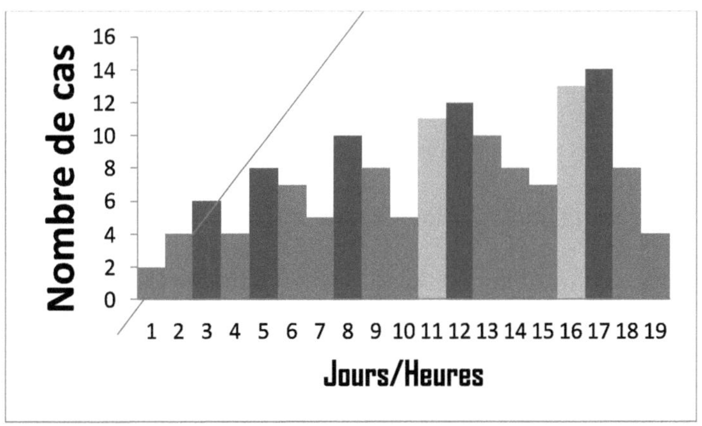

Example: Avian flu epidemic

5°) Calculate attack rates for different categories according to age, gender, occupation, etc.

6°) Identify the source and route of transmission: formulate hypotheses after establishing the transmission chain.

- What hypotheses might explain these data?
- Which is more likely?
- Why?
- How do you test this hypothesis?

7°) Test this (these) hypothesis(es) if necessary

8°) Carry out an environmental or biological survey if necessary

9°) Identify and apply appropriate control measures

- Preventive measures
- Treatment of infected persons

- Disseminate information on the epidemic to the public and healthcare workers.

10°) Complete analysis and epidemic investigation report

11°) Distribute these results

12°) Propose preventive measures

13°) Ensuring epidemiological surveillance

The objectives of the epidemic investigation are to :

- Confirm or deny the reality of the epidemic
- Formulate hypotheses concerning its origin (cause)
- Take curative and preventive measures

The survey is retrospective, as the epidemic has always been underway for several days, weeks or months, or has already ended.

7.1.4 How to determine whether an epidemic is present or not?

1. Identify the transmission level that represents an alarm threshold for initiating a

Investigation.

1.1 Establish criteria for initiating an investigation
1.2 Apply criteria for initiating an investigation

2. Verify or establish diagnosis for all known or suspected cases.

2.1 Establish case definition(s) (confirmed case, probable case, suspect case)

2.2 Confirm for all cases :

- That clinical examinations have been carried out,
- Whether or not the etiological agent has been identified,
- That appropriate diagnostic tests have been applied or are in progress,
- That the case definition criteria have been met.

3. Counting cases (preliminary count)

3.1 Define the information required and its source

3.2 Obtaining information

4. Define risk groups

4.1. Determine the distribution of cases in terms of time, place and person

4.2 Identifying the population from which cases originate

4.3. Calculate incidence rates (attack rates),

5. Determine whether the current incidence represents an epidemic or other situation requiring investigation.

7.1.5 How to characterize the epidemic?

1. Determine the information needed to characterize the epidemic in terms of time, place and person (with or without a diagnosis of certainty).

- Select person parameters (age, gender, profession, etc....)
- Select location parameters (home, school, workplace, etc.).
- Determine time of onset for all cases,
- Establishing an epidemic curve
- Obtain (or develop) the case investigation form.

2. Get information

2.1 Intensify the notification system (if necessary) or insist on new measures to introduce new measures for case identification and notification

2.2 Conduct interviews with clinicians, cases and contacts.

3. Organize data.

3.1 Identify criteria for grouping data appropriately

3.2 Calculate appropriate rates, ratios and proportions

3.3 Prepare tables, graphs and diagrams

4. Analyze and interpret data

4.1 Identify groups at risk in terms of time, people and place

4.2. Determining the incubation period

4.3 Determine the probable source and route of transmission.

7.1.6 How to prepare an epidemiological report

=> **Report elements**

- Introduction: problem statement, perspective (magnitude, who is affected, why is this problem important, data available), what is not known, reason/justification for the study.
- Methods/materials
  - ❖ Study population - how to select (number, sampling method)
  - ❖ Field methods (logistics, personnel, personnel training, travel, number of interviews/day, etc.)
  - ❖ Laboratory methods (if required)
  - ❖ Methods for data capture and analysis.
- Results

- Final sample (final population studied)
- Field conditions (if any problems)
- Analysis results (text, tables, graphs, etc.)

N.B.: no interpretation/judgment in the results section.

- Conclusions
  - Summarize key results (in less detail as a reminder)
  - Interpretation and explanation of these results.

The main aim of an epidemiological investigation of an epidemic is to identify measures to prevent ongoing transmission.

7.1.7 Investigating and declaring an epidemic

1. Investigation procedures

- Epidemiological reports - surveillance (hospital, C.S....)
- Rumors - from medical staff, the general public, daily observations...
- Limited epidemic: verbal report by someone involved or by medical staff treating cases (e.g. meningitis in the community, hepatitis A following a party, gastroenteritis, etc.).

2. The importance of epidemiological vigilance

- Don't miss out on an epidemic for which investigation (and possible intervention) is indicated.
- Harmful rumors: rumors of an epidemic (even false ones) can cause panic (false cases, false symptoms...) - especially in schools, among women.

3. Criteria for declaring an epidemic

- Verify the report with other sources of information - search at hospital level, CS, local practitioners (if necessary). Check diagnosis - what is the problem, what is it? For example: diarrhea = cholera, viral, etc. Vomiting = gastroenteritis, meningitis..., hemorrhagic fever, meningitis, ...
- Confirmation of the epidemic as the presence of an excessive number of cases (notion of normality and abnormality, endemic and pandemic) - use of past data (epidemiological curve, surveillance report, etc.).

7.2 EPIDEMIOLOGICAL SURVEILLANCE

7 .2.1 Definition

It's a process that involves the ongoing study of individuals, environmental elements and the agent of disease or health-related phenomena in the community, regardless of the severity of the epidemiological situation. Its aim is to prevent the emergence of new epidemics.

According to Thackers et al, epidemiological surveillance is the systematic and continuous collection, analysis and interpretation of health data for use in the planning, implementation and evaluation of public health practices. It is the collection of health data to support decision-making and public health action.

The U.S. Centers for Disease Control and Prevention (CDC) have defined epidemiological surveillance as a systematic and continuous process of collecting, analyzing and interpreting health data essential to the planning, implementation and evaluation of public health programs, closely linked to the rapid dissemination of these data to key stakeholders.

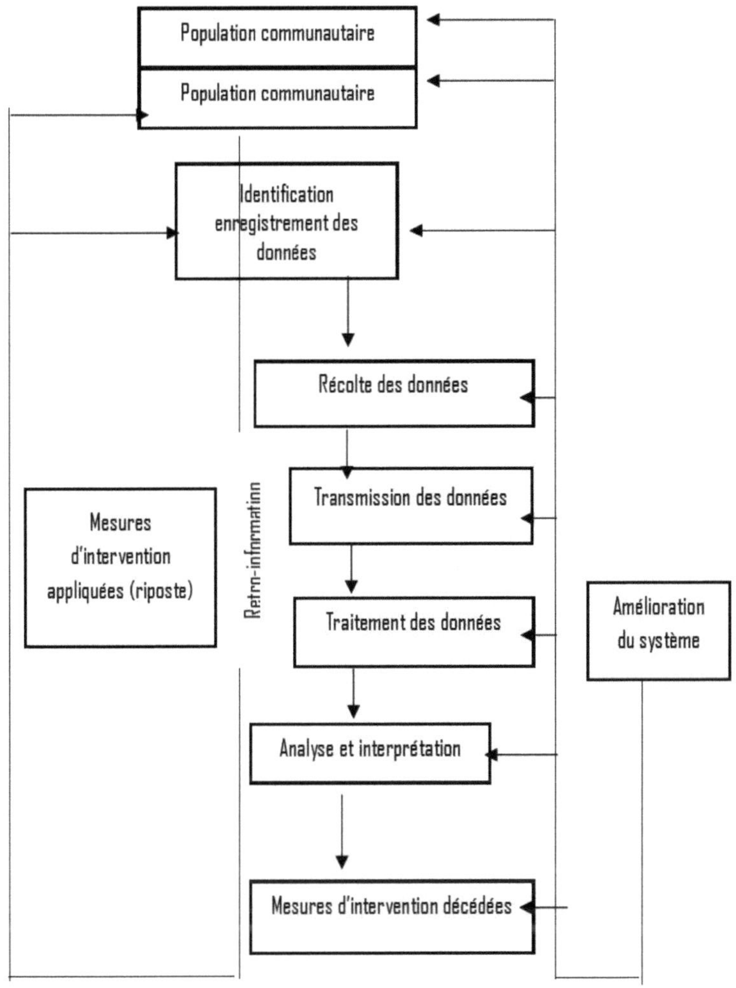

Case detection, data collection and reporting, data organization and analysis, investigation and feedback, information dissemination and response are the core activities of epidemiological surveillance.

Health problems that warrant epidemiological surveillance are those with a significant health or social impact: high frequency, severity, possible transmission to others, high social cost, etc.

The design of a surveillance system varies from country to country. In the Democratic Republic of Congo, the mechanism for collecting health data begins at the health center (health post), which transmits the data to the health zone, the health zone transmits the data to the health district, and the health district in turn transmits the data to the provincial health inspectorate (4ème office). Each province is expected to transmit statistics to the central 4ème Directorate. At each level, the information must be checked and corrective action taken.

There is also a sentinel system for reporting and monitoring a number of target diseases.

The data collected forms an important basis for planning health programs, and for the control, monitoring and evaluation of control and prevention activities.

7.2.2 Practical aims of epidemiological surveillance

Epidemiological surveillance has the following practical aims:

- Facilitate the planning, execution and control of anti-epidemic and preventive measures;
- The ability to react rapidly to changes in the epidemiological situation (early warning system);
- Maintain productivity and reduce absenteeism;
- Predicting the development of the epidemiological situation;
- Leading basic and applied research;
- Develop standard work and uniform, comparable methods.

Epidemiological surveillance thus makes it possible to :

- Estimate the importance of health problems in order to plan the resources to be allocated to their prevention and management, taking priorities into account;
- Tracking temporal and spatial trends ;
- Early detection of changes in infectious and non-infectious agents;
- Improve knowledge of vectors and modes of disease transmission;
- Detecting knowledge about vectors and modes of disease transmission ;
- Early detection and monitoring of epidemics or abnormal phenomena;
- Sound the alarm and organize the response;
- Suggest hypotheses regarding the emergence of a health problem or a change in the trend of a problem at risk;
- Apply control and management measures to reduce incidence and lethality;
- Evaluate preventive measures ;
- Evaluate the effectiveness of disease management or identify changes in management;
- Plan interventions and improve professional practices.

This continuous process enables us to rapidly detect and act on changes in the appearance and distribution of diseases or health problems.

Monitoring allows us to sound the alarm and take action.

7.2.3 Areas to be monitored

The spectrum of information to be collected includes the following elements:

- Individual characteristics ;
- The external environment and interventions affecting health

We are therefore interested in :

- Illness or other health problems: How many cases? How many deaths?
- The person: who gets sick? who dies? (age, gender)
- Location: where the disease occurs: living quarters, travel, etc.
- The moment: when? for how long?
- The how: mode of transmission, disease expression, onset signs, state period, terminal stage and etiological factors.

Monitoring methods are based on :

- A mandatory reporting system for certain communicable diseases;
- Data from healthcare and laboratory activities;
- Data specifically collected within the framework of registers on a defined geographical basis;
- Regular periodic surveys of general population samples.

Epidemiological surveillance can cover the following areas:

1. Regular notification of deaths or ongoing study of mortality and morbidity

- Study of morbidity measured by the following indicators:
  Incidence: new cases

  Prevalence: old and new cases.

- Study of mortality and lethality by age, gender, cause of death, etc.

2. Serological surveillance and serosurveillance

It consists of looking for serological indicators of contact between the infectious agent and a receptive site. This contact is generally marked by the presence of specific antibodies against the infectious agent in question. In the case of diseases or infections that confer lasting protective immunity, serosurveillance can be used to establish the degree of herd immunity. The concept of herd immunity is a very important one in public health, particularly in the epidemiology of infectious diseases, because it indicates the number of individuals already resistant to the disease, forming a barrier to the spread of infection in the exposed general population.

3. Biotope monitoring

This involves regular analysis of the situation of natural germ reservoirs.

4. Monitoring biological interactions

Study ecological changes and monitor the identification of new germs appearing in a population.

7.2.4 Monitoring stages

Epidemiological surveillance is a process based on :

1. Morbidity and mortality data collection + etiological factors
2. Data formatting and presentation
3. Data analysis and interpretation
4. Disseminating this data

5. Use of these data to implement control measures and provide feedback

The following steps should be followed:

1. Establish objectives and determine the data to be collected (indicators) ;
2. Data collection ;
3. Analyze and interpret data ;
4. Formulating etiological hypotheses ;
5. Testing hypotheses ;
6. Recommend or implement control measures ;
7. Prepare and distribute the report (feedback) ;
8. Evaluate the monitoring system, i.e. whether or not objectives have been achieved.

1. Collecting data :

Methods :

- Outpatient register
- Inpatient and outpatient files
- Scorecard

Types of data to be collected :

- Disease (operational case definition required)
- Profession
- Age, religion, address, socio-economic level, etc.

2. Data compilation

- Drawing up disease tables
- Present data in diagrams, histograms, maps, etc.

3. Data analysis

- Identify groups most affected, seasonal variations, etc.
- Calculate notification rates by province.

4. Preventive measures based on analysis results

5. Data declaration: Notify promptly.

Zero or null report" transmission: notify even if there are no cases, i.e. report 0 cases. Always keep one or more copies of the notification.

6. Feedback

Feedback is very important in epidemiological surveillance for a variety of reasons, including motivating field staff and assessing its effectiveness. Feedback also serves to disseminate information and to encourage staff who carry out regular surveillance.

7. In the event of an epidemiological emergency: assess the need for an epidemiological investigation prior to data reporting, and conduct the investigation according to a standardized scheme.

(Epidemiological emergency = ==> Investigation)

1. *Proving the reality of the epidemic;*
2. *Check the diagnosis of the suspected disease;*
3. *Establish criteria for identifying cases of the disease;*
4. *Identify cases ;*
5. *Describe the epidemiological situation in terms of time, place and people affected;*
6. *Summarize and analyze the information gathered and formulate hypotheses to explain the epidemiological situation;*
7. *Check assumptions ;*

8. *Develop preventive actions and control strategies ;*
9. *Evaluate the effectiveness and efficiency of the control strategy.*
10. *Write a report on the epidemic;*
11. *Research the disease and its control measures.*

7.2.5 Types of monitoring systems

1. Passive surveillance

The monitoring system is dependent on the cooperation of the care services, which are supposed to report on a routine basis. Often, health-care providers do not feel obliged to report. This type of monitoring is nevertheless the most common approach; its weaknesses are lack of completeness and promptness.

2. Active monitoring

The surveillance system takes the initiative in contacting care facilities to collect data. The data is of better quality, and generally more timely and complete. Unfortunately, this approach is costly and time-consuming. Hence, it is only applied to specific diseases, such as disease eradication or elimination.

3. Sentinel surveillance

A surveillance system can be sentinel when it targets specific sites and groups. For example, HIV surveillance may target pregnant women attending antenatal clinics. It may also target young people attending STI consultations, etc.....

Sentinel surveillance can select a site and then monitor the health care facilities serving that site. For example, choroquine resistance surveillance in 2000-2001 was carried out in Kimpese, Kapolowe, Mikkkoyi, Bukavu, Vanga, Kisangani, Lutshuru and Kingasani.

Sentinel surveillance is the type of surveillance where certain sites meeting precise criteria are selected to provide information on the evolution of disease or infectious state in a given population or group of people. The sites selected are generally medical facilities whose reports are particularly reliable in providing indications of the health situation in their provinces.

- Passive data collected on certain sites
- Selected sites
- Selection criteria: geographical, reliability (regularity, quality)
- Sometimes requires more training, supervision.

4. **Routine monitoring**

This type of surveillance is based on passive data collection at the level of the entire healthcare system. Passive data is normally collected to look for trends. It is data that already exists/is available; it is data collected that is not based on the general population. Information is often given only on the number of cases (often not specified by age, sex, vaccination status, etc.).

5. General surveillance (exhaustive surveillance)

This type of surveillance concerns the entire population.

6. Case-by-case monitoring.

This type of surveillance implies that for each suspected case of a given disease, an investigation is carried out to find out how the disease occurred.

The diagnosis will be confirmed by a laboratory test.

7. Community-based surveillance

Community leaders or community health workers trained in the diagnosis of certain diseases can act as contacts for the screening of suspected cases and their notification to the facilities.

The activities to be carried out at community level are as follows:

1. Notify the nearest health facilities of cases covered by community-based surveillance:
2. Assist community health workers in the investigation of cases/outbreaks of disease;
3. Use the information provided by community health workers to make decisions, particularly on health education and the coordination of community participation in disease control.

8. Integrated monitoring

It's a surveillance strategy that targets all diseases declared under surveillance in the country, by pooling resources to combat them.

9. Vertical monitoring

This type of monitoring is usually carried out by specialized programs. Here, monitoring activities are specific to the program, and resources are not shared with other programs.

GENERAL CONCLUSION

Epidemiology remains an indispensable tool for public health research and informed decision-making. The integration of theoretical concepts, understanding of causality and modern practices enables researchers and decision-makers to better understand disease dynamics and develop effective responses. As new challenges emerge, such as emerging infectious diseases and chronic disease issues, it is crucial to maintain a rigorous and evolving approach to epidemiology.

The aim of this book is to lay the foundations for critical thinking, and to guide the reader in the practical application of this knowledge.

BIBLIOGRAPHY

1. Ancelle T. Statistique Epidémiologie, Maloine, 2006
2. André Simpson & Clément Beau. Epidemiologie initiation à la lecture critique en sciences de la santé 3ème edition (Québec)
3. Anny Robert, Quantitative epidemiology, UCL, 2010
4. Beaglehole R, Bonita R and Kjellström T: Eléments d'épidémiologie, WHO Geneva, 1994
5. Beaucage C, Bonnier Viger Y. Epidémiologie appliquée, Editions Gaëtan Morin, 1996.
6. Bernard JM and Lapointe C: Mesures statistiques en épidémiologie, Québec, Presses de l'Université du Québec, 1991
7. Czernickow P. Chaperon J, Le Couteur X: Epidemiology: knowledge and practice. Masson, Paris 2001
8. Dabis F, Drucker J and Moren A. Epidemiology of intervention, Aenztte 1992
9. Dean T. Jamison, Joel G. Breman, Anthony R. Measham, Gearges Alleyne, Mariam Claeson, David B, Evans, Prabhat Jha, Anne Mills, Philip Musgrove. Health priorities: World Bank, Washington, 2006
10. Deghome, Epidemiology in the field, UCL, 2010
11. Dilhuydy, M.H. Benefit and cost of cervical screening. Gynecology, 1987, Quebec
12. Gordis Leon. Epidemiology: Fourth Edition. Saunders Elsevier, 2008
13. Guide technique pour la surveillance intégrée de la maladie et riposte, 4ème direction / direction de la lutte contre la maladie, in press 2011
14. Hennekens, C,H,J,E Buring ET S.L Maynentac, Epidemiology in medicine, Paris, Frison - Roche, 1998

15. http. ://en.wikipedia.org/w/index.php,demographic transition
16. Jenick M and Cléroux R: Epidemiology: Principles, Techniques, Applications, Quebec, Edisem Inc and Maloïne S.A, 1984
17. Landrivon G : Delahaye F : Clinical research. From idea to publication. Masson, 1995
18. Mac Mahon B. Trichopoulos D: Epidemiology. Princiaples & Méthods, Boston/Toronto: Little, Brown and Company, 1996
19. MATUKALA, Epidemiology CESO, ISTM - Kinshasa, 2018
20. Minerva : Revue d'Evidence Based Medicine (http://www.minerva-ebm.be/).
21. Moyes Szklo and Javier Nieto F: Epidemiology Beyond the basics, An aspen publication 2000
22. WHO; Integrated epidemiological surveillance, Geneva, 1998
23. R. Knafou, Les hommes et la terre, Géographie 2e , éd, belin, 1996
24. Rothman KJ, Greenland S: Modem epidemiology, Philadelphia. Lippincott-Raven Publishers, 1998
25. Rumeau - Rouquette C, Blonde B, Kamiski Met Bréart G: Epidemiology methods and practice, Médecine - Sciences, Flammarion, 1993
26. Health economics & medical information processing (https://sesstim.univ-amu.fr/fr/page/glossaire-epidemiologie-et-recherche-medicale)
27. Tonglet R.: Notes de cours d'épidémiologie, Cercle Médical Saint-luc, 2001

Sumário

APPENDICES

APPENDIX 1: PRACTICAL EXERCISES

Question .1. . Which association measure to use :

a) in an "open" survey where workers exposed or not to asbestos are followed and the occurrence of cancer is measured?

b) in a food-borne illness?

c) C) when you want to identify risk factors for a rare disease?

Question .2. Between 1966 and 1969, Herbest and Cully identified seven cases of clear-cell carcinoma of the vagina in girls under 22 years of age in the Boston area. At that time, the same number of cases were reported in the international literature.

a) what type of study was needed to understand the origin of the problem? Justify in two (2) lines

b) Mothers' exposure to distilbene (a synthetic estrogen prescribed to pregnant women in case of threatened spontaneous abortion) has been identified as the almost exclusive risk factor for cancer in these young women.

What method would you suggest for measuring the extent of the phenomenon (measuring the incidence or prevalence of this type of cancer)?

Question .1. Consider a city with 8700 inhabitants per km2. Assume that :

. An infected individual moves an average of 0.001 km2 per day.

. The probability of infection transmission (given contact) is 40%.

. A person is "infectious" for six days before becoming immune.

a. *What model will you use to describe this?*
b. *How will the evolution of infected individuals change if a person is "infectious" for only 2 days before becoming immune?*

Question .1. What is the maximum proportion of unvaccinated people that a fully susceptible population can support without risking an epidemic in the case of the introduction of a disease with OR equal to 5 :

(a) If the vaccine is 100% effective.
(b) If the vaccine is 80% effective.
Answer (only for Q 10 and Q 11)
a. Necessary protection = P 1-1/RO =1/5=8=80%.
b. P=vaccination*Effectiveness - Vaccination=protection /Effectiveness=80%=1=100%.

Question .1. The probability of being infected with influenza is 0.20 per year. What percentage of children have been in contact with the virus at least once by the age of six?

Question .1. Ninety percent of a school population of 7558 pupils were vaccinated against whooping cough. There were 836 cases of pertussis during the year, including 455 among those vaccinated.
How would you respond to the following table?

Why aren't cohort studies the most appropriate way to study rare diseases such as certain cancers?

Question .1. In a hospital ward, 3 cases of MRSA were reported in 2 weeks. Fearing that the patients had been infected by the same person, it was decided to analyze the distribution of affected patients by nursing staff. It was found that 2 nurses had cared for all 3 MRSA patients. After microbiological analysis, it was concluded that one of the 2 nurses was MRSA-positive and could be the source of the infection at the hospital.

a. what type of study was used?

b. why is this type of study the most appropriate?

Question .1. 15. The Kibondo district in Tanzania is home to 170,000 Burundian refugees in 4 camps. Between March 2000 and May 2001 (inclusive, i.e. 15 months), these 4 refugee camps were hit by a measles epidemic. The number of cases per camp was :

Camp number of cases
Kanembwa 10
Karago 739
Mtendeli 93
Nduta 220

c) Mtendeli
d) Nduta
e) Impossible to caculate

Question .2. You want to study the difference in road deaths between men and women. How do you define case groups?

a) The group of men who died as a result of a road accident;
b) The group of men and women who died as a result of a road accident;
c) the group of men and women who died of all causes;
d) the men's group.

Question .3. You' re studying the relationship between an exposure factor X and mortality in a population of men and women. Here are your data:

Presentations: 80

30 deceased: 10 men, 20 women

50 living people: 20 men, 30 women

Unexposed: 120

45 deceased: 20 men, 25 women

75 living: 10 men, 65 women

Calculate the RR and what is your conclusion?

Question .4. A research center wants to study the effect of beer on the incidence of heart attacks.

a) Case definition? Those who have suffered a heart attack

b) Definition of exposure ? Beer consumption

C) type of study ? Cohort

d) OR or RR? RR

e) Possible biases?

Describe how you intend to undertake this study.

CONTRIBUTIONS FROM

This research is part of an in-depth study carried out after several observations and surveys in certain provinces of the Democratic Republic of Congo (DRC), and our experience in research and teaching, which we have used throughout the researcher has indeed contributed its share in the elaboration and publication of this book.

Our thanks go to AG Alexis TOHEMO LUKAMBA (tohemoalexisluka6@gmail.com), National Coordinator of the Centre de recherche et de promotion en Gestion des institutions de santé (CERPROGIS ASBL, in French), who finalized text processing and some computer work.

CONFLICTS OF INTEREST

The author declares no conflict of interest in this study, as no funder or respondent played a leading role in the interpretation of the study results.

No one was forced to take part in the study, and the information provided was used solely for the purposes of this study. The writing of the manuscript and the decision to publish it were the sole responsibility of the author.

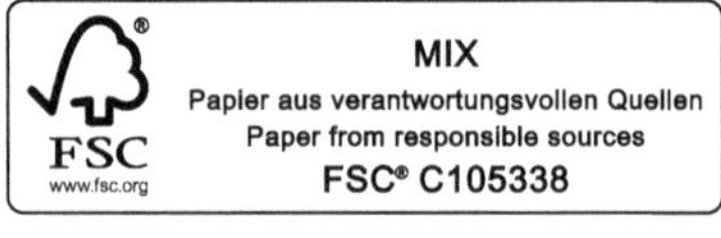

Printed by Books on Demand GmbH, Norderstedt / Germany